Talking with Patients about the
Personal Impact of Illness

Talking with Patients about the Personal Impact of Illness

The Doctor's Role

LENORE M. BUCKLEY, MD, MPH
Professor of Internal Medicine and Pediatrics
Virginia Commonwealth University
School of Medicine

Foreword by
ARTHUR W. FRANK, PhD
Professor, Department of Sociology
University of Calgary
Canada

Radcliffe Publishing
Oxford • New York

Radcliffe Publishing Ltd
18 Marcham Road
Abingdon
Oxon OX14 1AA
United Kingdom

www.radcliffe-oxford.com
Electronic catalogue and worldwide online ordering facility.

British Library Cataloguing in Publication Data

A catalogue record for this book is available from the British Library.

ISBN-13: 978 184619 289 0

Typeset by Pindar New Zealand, Auckland, New Zealand
Printed and bound by TJI Digital, Padstow, Cornwall, UK

Contents

Foreword

THE TWO PHYSICIANS IN THE TREATMENT ROOM

Much is written about patient-centered care and the patient experience. What sets this book apart is, first, Lenore Buckley's ability to tell stories about her own medical experience. These teaching tales give young physicians a sense of the task that their profession requires of them, while keeping that task within human proportions. Second and complementing that is her excellent compilation of quotations and stories from the memoirs of patients and physicians, especially physicians as patients. Here Dr. Buckley as author models the clinical skill she recommends: remaining quiet and letting the patient speak.

As I read this compilation of resources for young physicians and their teachers, two questions occurred to me. On the patient side, what do I want from my physician? And on the physician side, what do I expect from myself?

Patients, in my experience of being one and of talking to many others, want two physicians to be present in the treatment room. One is the treatment expert, who will make the correct diagnosis, know the best referral, or prescribe the most effective medication. The treatment expert has to get it right: right diagnosis, right intervention. The other doctor in the room is the witness to the suffering of illness. For the witness, there is no single right response; the most meaningful response may be respectful silence.

Witnessing begins with allowing oneself to see the widest scope of what is happening; not simply the diagnostic signs and the responses to treatment, but also the extensive suffering that illness brings into lives. As Dr. Buckley points out, illness affects not only the life of the patient, but also the broader circle of caregivers, including family and friends. Willingness to see is the beginning. The next part is recognition: communicating what is seen in a way that helps people to *hold their own*, because that is much of what living with suffering is, holding one's own. Recognition is based on a simple, three-part message: I see your suffering; I honour your living with this suffering; I respect that it is an achievement to live as you must, with your illness.

That brings us to the physician's question: what do I expect of myself? Or, responding to the patient's need: can I call myself a physician and not be both expert and witness? Lest this question seem overwhelming, I have good news for physicians: most patients are willing to be generous in their expectations. Patients know full well that physicians have limited resources, beginning with time. Most patients, all but a few, do not expect their physicians to become healers of their lives, any more than they expect medical miracles. They do expect that physicians will see what they are living with, honor their efforts to live as best they can, and give them credit for the achievement that each day is. This recognition *need not take much time*: a simple pause, holding eye contact, can communicate a depth of recognition, when done at the right moment. The timing takes practice, and if the young physician is lucky, a good role model helps.

Dr. Buckley offers physicians some very good questions that will allow them to expand their vision and understanding of their patients' lives. A book of this size necessarily says less about what to do after patients actually answer those questions, telling the physician exactly how hard their lives are. An old clinical rule is that whatever a clinician opens up, she or he has a responsibility to address. Keeping this rule in mind, my advice to physicians is to be realistic in how you ask the recommended questions. If you know your time is limited, preface the question with something like: "There may not be much I can do to help, but as I try to care for you, it would be valuable for me to know. . ." That introductory phrasing cues the patient that the physician does care, but also that the physician's response may be limited. When patients have spoken – without being interrupted – physicians can again be realistic, first pausing for a moment of recognition, then thanking the patient for opening his or her life in this way, and finally asking what they could do to help, either themselves or by recommending other resources. Very often, patients will simply express gratitude for the physician's willingness to listen. Patients are grateful, in part because they want to believe their physicians care.

I hope this empathic, useful collection of materials for teaching and reflection finds its way into medical school curricula, and I hope it is one of those books that physicians return to during years of practice, especially when they sense that the treatment expert is crowding the witness out of the room. Patients need both doctors. Lenore Buckley shows how doctors are able to expect nothing less of themselves.

Arthur W. Frank, PhD
Professor, Department of Sociology
University of Calgary
Canada
June 2008

Preface

I grew up in a family affected by chronic illness and, before my medical training, I had the chance to spend time with family members at their visits to the doctor and during hospitalizations. Early on, I was aware of the awkwardness of the conversations between patients and their physicians, and I was especially aware of what was never said. There seemed to be reluctance on both sides to discuss the impact of the illness on their life and future, to talk about their fears, and to discuss how they were coping and what to expect, day to day.

When I was in the first year of medical school, I accompanied my mother to a routine doctor's appointment. My mother did her medical training during World War II, married and had a family, and continued to practice well into her sixties. To this day, she is the most determined, optimistic, and resourceful person I have known. Despite all of her knowledge, personal strength, and connections, she struggled to deal with the profound changes in her life when she went into renal failure in her early fifties.

On that particular day, while we waited in the clinic examination room, she joked about the article in a dialysis newsletter about making Christmas decorations out of old plastic dialysate bottles. Then, after a few quiet moments, she told me for the first time that she was exhausted and afraid. She was not sure how long she would be able to go on living on dialysis, which was a relatively new procedure at the time, and she was worried about the future, potential complications, and changes in her roles now that she was dependent on other people.

Minutes later, when her doctor whisked into the room and asked how she was doing, my mother perked up, smiled, and told him she was fine.

Fine? I looked over at her, confused. It was clear that she was not fine but, somehow, my mother could not bring herself to tell her doctor. There was a short discussion of medications and blood tests, and we were done. Over the 20 years he cared for her, my mother and her doctor talked about her children – where they all went to school, who married, and who had children. But, as far as I know, he never asked her how she was coping with a devastating illness, and my mother never brought it up.

I left the visit that day feeling confused, deflated, and disappointed. Although, at the time, I didn't understand the impact of the illness on her life, I did have the feeling that something important, even momentous, was happening to her and that she was struggling to understand it and to reorganize her life to deal with it. I also had the feeling that her doctor was concerned about her well-being and aware of her struggle, but he either didn't know what to say to help or didn't think it was part of his job to say it. However, if he didn't help her to understand the challenges in the road that lay ahead, and what living with this illness would be like, who would?

Some would say that my mother just had the bad luck to have doctors with poor interpersonal skills, or that it was a different era in medicine. However, I think it was more than that. She had a competent, even caring physician, and there were countless visits to other doctors over the years where the conversation was essentially the same – factual, informational, and impersonal. I think, in retrospect, that those well-meaning doctors had absolutely no idea what to say. They were trained in the pathophysiology and treatment of disease, but they didn't understand what it was like to live with the illness. It was not part of their personal experience or their training.

I don't think I completely understood this issue until 20 years later, when I was the attending physician on a general medicine service. We had admitted a pleasant, undemanding, and soft-spoken 40-year-old man to our service for treatment of pneumonia. He was the local postmaster in a very small, rural Virginia town – a town in which he had grown up, and where he knew and interacted with everyone. After a 6-month work up for fatigue and weight loss, his family physician checked an HIV test and it was positive. Surprised, he checked it again. It was positive again and the CD4 count was low. Mr. Phillips was referred to our HIV clinic where his treatment was begun. However, months later, he continued to lose weight and to be readmitted for one infection after another. Now he was admitted to our service.

It was the medical student who first noticed that he was depressed. While we were busy ordering medications, doing tests, and getting consultants involved, he had spent the most time talking with the patient. After a few days, he came into the team room and asked, almost embarrassed, if he could talk to me. "I just don't know what to say to Mr. Phillips." He went on to explain that Mr. Phillips told him that he didn't care if he got better, and admitted that he was not taking his HIV medications. After filling prescriptions at the local pharmacy, his diagnosis of HIV/AIDS quickly became public knowledge in his home town. Given the stigma of the illness in this community, he felt that he could never return to his previous job and that even continuing to live in town with his mother, in the place where he had been well known and well liked, was not an option – for his mother's sake as well as for his.

"I just don't feel that I know enough to offer him any advice. I can't imagine how difficult this is for him", the medical student said, recognizing that something significant was happening.

I was struck that day by the distress of this student, who could empathize with Mr. Phillips but didn't know what to say or where to start. And, as I listened to him, I thought back over my own medical training. When *do* doctors learn what to say in this situation? Was it just his inexperience? Would time and the example of supervising physicians fill in the gaps in his knowledge in this area, just as we expect they will fill in the gaps in his clinical skills and judgment? I couldn't remember anyone ever discussing the physician's role in educating and counseling patients about living with serious illness. And observations of more senior trainees and attending physicians don't necessarily validate the assumption that we reliably learn this by example. Doctors are not known for their ability to talk to patients about the personal impact of illness.

This book is written for all physicians, but is directed particularly to medical students and trainees. If some of the most devastating aspects of serious illness are uncertainty, vulnerability, and loss of control, then medical training is a perfect "teaching moment" to discuss the personal aspects of illness. As you start your clinical rotations, medical students and trainees must learn a new language, a new kind of problem solving, and take on new roles with responsibility and culpability. You are thrown on to the hospital floors and into the lives of seriously ill patients with an education that supplies only the very basic information and survival skills that you will need. Making mistakes, not knowing the answers, and feeling inadequate are part of everyday life. As you move from rotation to rotation, expectations are sometimes unclear, you don't have control over your daily routine, and the new and unfamiliar world that you have entered can feel overwhelming. Students and residents understand vulnerability, uncertainty, and lack of control, and sometimes feel isolated from the person they were and the friends and life that they had before they submerged themselves in medical training.

So this is an ideal time to stop and think about the impact of vulnerability, uncertainty, isolation, and lack of control on the personal lives of those who are seriously ill. The truth is that most of us feel inadequately prepared for the job as we start our clinical training. It is an apprenticeship, and the majority of what we need to know is learned "on the job" and by example. So the example of supervising physicians is critically important for the development of skills in discussing the psychosocial impact of illness with patients. No matter what you are taught in the first 2 years of medical school about open-ended questions, humanism, ethics, and the impact of illness, most physicians learn from the behavior of supervising and attending physicians during training. If, in the fast-moving culture of clinical medicine, the most respected physicians model empathic behavior, talk about the psychosocial impact of illness, and set high expectations about doctor–patient interactions, students learn this by example. If psychosocial issues are never discussed or are left to nurses and social workers, then we learn that this is not "doctor's work", and often continue that way of interacting with patients for the rest of our career.

This book explores the psychosocial impact of serious illness and the doctor's role in counseling patients. Even the most seasoned physician often feels at a loss to know what to say to a distressed patient who is struggling with the personal aspects of serious illness and disability. It is not something we are routinely taught. It takes time, attention, and skill. Most physicians who are good at this learn what to say from observations of physicians whom they respect and the conversations that they share with patients over many years of practice. Our patients become our teachers. Like everything else in medicine, there is a continuous learning curve. This book offers a beginning.

Lenore M. Buckley
June 2008

About the Author

Dr. Lenore Buckley is an adult and pediatric rheumatologist specializing in the care of chronic illnesses such as rheumatoid arthritis, lupus, and other autoimmune diseases. She is a Professor of Medicine and Pediatrics at the Virginia Commonwealth University School of Medicine in Richmond, Virginia, a member of the Board of Directors and the Public Health Council of the Arthritis Foundation in the USA, and a former member of the board of directors of the American College of Rheumatology. Dr. Buckley teaches a senior seminar to medical students on the psychosocial aspects of chronic illness, and is a recipient of the Robert S. Irby Award for Volunteer Leadership from the Virginia Arthritis Foundation and the Clinician of the Year Award from the Virginia Commonwealth University clinical faculty in 2006.

Acknowledgments

This book is a compilation of the thoughts, experiences, and reflections of many people who have lived with and thought carefully about the personal impact of serious illness. These writers had the courage to reveal very personal aspects of their own experience, and were gracious enough to let me use their work in this book.

I want to thank the many patients for whom I have had the privilege of caring, some for just a few minutes and some for decades. Years of conversation and laughter about issues great and small gave me invaluable insights about how people cope with illness. They will always have my gratitude and respect.

Wei Ming Hsu worked with me from the beginning of the project, combining the text and images into a graphic layout that maximized their impact and meaning. Dr. Curt Sessler provided the wonderful photography. Betty Dodson coordinated the project with patience and humor. Joanna Roberts provided editorial assistance.

Finally, I would like to thank my family: my father, who has patiently listened to and counseled me for decades; my mother, who showed me how to combine the roles of mother, spouse, friend, physician, and patient with grace and humor; my brothers and sisters, who are always there to offer advice and help; my husband, who provided years of support and encouragement; and my children, who are my inspiration and are proud of my work, even when it takes time away from them.

List of Permissions

Excerpts from *A Whole New Life: an illness and a healing* by Reynolds Price reprinted with permission of Scribner, an imprint of Simon & Schuster Adult Publishing Group.

Excerpts from *Local Wonders: seasons in the Bohemian Alps* by Ted Kooser by permission of the University of Nebraska Press. © 2002

Excerpts from *The Nature of Suffering and the Goals of Medicine* by Eric Cassel by permission of Oxford University Press. © 1991

Excerpts from *At the Will of the Body: reflections on illness* by Arthur Frank and Catherine E Foote reprinted by permission of Houghton Mifflin Harcourt Publishing Company. All rights reserved. © 1991

Excerpts from *Empathy and the Practice of Medicine*, edited by Howard Spiro *et al.* reprinted by permission of Yale University Press. © 1993

Excerpts from *The Youngest Science*: *Notes of a Medicine Watcher* by Lewis Thomas by permission of the Penguin Group. All rights reserved. © 1983

*To my mother
who is my anchor.*

. . . Medicine has done well with my body, and I am grateful. But doing with the body is only part of what needs to be done for the person. What happens when my body breaks down happens not just to my body but also my life, which is lived in that body. When the body breaks down, so does the life. Even when medicine can fix the body, it doesn't always put the life back together again. Medicine can diagnose and treat the breakdown, but sometimes so much fear and frustration have been aroused in the ill person that fixing the breakdown does not quiet them. At those times, the experience of illness goes beyond the limits of medicine.

Arthur Frank, PhD

Introduction

Education about death and dying has become an important and routine part of medical training. Most students receive specific instruction about end-of-life care, the impact of terminal illness on the patient and their family, and resources for support and counseling. However, as treatments for life-threatening diseases improve, many people with serious diseases are not dying. They are living with chronic conditions that may make their life more physically limited and uncertain. So it may be time to ask the question: Are we adequately training physicians to educate and counsel patients about the significant personal impact of serious illness on their life?

Personal responses to illness are strongly affected by an individual's personality – their innate optimism or pre-existing tendency to anxiety or depression. However, regardless of personality, few people are prepared for the profound changes in personal life that come with illness. The challenges are surprisingly similar across different diseases – cancer, organ failure, autoimmune disease, physical disability, and chronic infections. These serious illnesses lead to vulnerability, uncertainty, lack of control, isolation, and enormous changes in self-image and self-esteem.

A person's roles – both personal and professional – change dramatically during serious illness. Patients struggle to understand these changes and to find resources to help them rebuild their life, their self-image, and their self-esteem. Most are successful, but some never fully recover a life that is acceptable to them. They continue to mourn for the life they might have lived and the things they might have done if it were not for the physical, psychological, and financial impact of illness. Even those who do recover often find that their life or their outlook on life has been permanently changed.

What is surprising is that most physicians and healthcare providers are relatively unaware of the potentially devastating effects of severe illness on the patient's personal life. There are a number of barriers to this understanding. Because of improvements in the prevention and treatment of diseases over the last 50 years, many doctors have had little or no personal experience of illness. And, during medical school or residency, most have received little instruction about the psychosocial aspects of illness. We learn about how to discuss illness with patients by watching more senior physicians during training, but this type of learning can be haphazard and incomplete. Time is also an obstacle. The hectic pace of training and medical practice does not leave much time for leisurely conversation with patients about their personal life and family that would give us insights about the impact of the illness on the person.

And, the most important barrier may be the differences between the lives of physicians and those of the seriously ill patients whom they treat. Doctors are well educated, generally financially secure, and are often younger than the people they care for. Physical and financial well-being makes them relatively independent – they have the power and resources to choose a direction in life. To patients, they appear to be in control of their lives – both physically and financially. However, people who are facing a serious illness often feel the opposite – vulnerable, uncertain about their future, and dependent on family and friends for help, and on physicians and medical personnel for treatment.

These differences in power, control, and vulnerability create a psychological divide between physicians and patients. Many doctors are unaware of it, and many patients never try to cross it. They won't raise personal issues with their doctor, either because they assume that the doctor just wouldn't understand, or because they don't want to appear vulnerable in front of a doctor who appears to be very much in control. As patients form relationships with their physicians, they often want to be seen as a competent person and a "good" patient. They may worry that questions about psychosocial issues will make them look weak, complaining, or ungrateful.

Some people are simply embarrassed by their normal emotional response to illness, such as anxiety, anger, or depression. So these conversations are saved for people with whom they are more comfortable – the nurse, family members, close friends, or other people who have experienced a serious illness. Or they may never occur at all.

Interviews with practicing physicians reveal that the humanistic and personal interactions which they have with patients enrich their careers in medicine. In 1998, the Association of American Medical Colleges (AAMC) identified four essential attributes to be considered in the education of medical students – altruism, knowledge, skill, and duty. In defining altruism, they state:

> Physicians must be compassionate and empathetic in caring for patients, and must be trustworthy in all professional dealings. They must bring to the study of medicine those character traits, attitudes, and values that underpin ethical and beneficent medical care. They must understand the history of medicine, the nature of medicine's social compact, the ethical precepts of the medical profession, and their obligations under law. At all times they must act with integrity, honesty, and respect for patients' privacy and respect for the dignity of patients as persons. In all of their interactions with patients, they must seek to understand the meaning of the patients' stories in the context of the patients' beliefs and family and cultural values.
>
> *Association of American Medical Colleges*

Studies tell us that the physicians who are best able to understand the psychosocial impact of illness are often those who have been ill themselves, or who have had a close friend or family member who was ill. That experience gives them an understanding of how a person's life is changed by illness and, supported and motivated by that knowledge, they are better able to discuss these issues with their patients.

One way to help doctors to understand the patient's experience is through personal memoirs about illness – especially those of physicians, with whom they naturally identify. This book includes numerous passages written by people who have had a serious illness, including Dr. Fitzhugh Mullan's memoir about his treatment for seminoma, Dr. Kay Redfield Jamison's story about her life and career with manic-depressive illness, the insights of Dr. Arthur Frank (a medical sociologist) about the impact of myocarditis and testicular cancer on his life and career, and poet and author Reynolds Price's memoir about his treatment for spinal cord cancer. Other sources used for this book include a discussion of the doctor–patient relationship in *Medicine as a Human Experience* by Drs. Reiser and Rosen, Dr. Arthur Kleinman's book about the impact of illness, *The Illness Narratives: Suffering, Healing, and the Human Condition*, and physicians' essays about what they learned from their own illness from the *Annals of Internal Medicine* and the book *When Doctors Get Sick* by Drs. Mandell and Spiro.

The "voices" of these people make the experience of illness more personal and tangible. Their narratives allow us to step into their shoes and understand how day-to-day life, relationships, and goals are changed by serious illness.

In the introduction to *A Life in Medicine: a Literary Anthology*, Dr. Robert Coles reminds us that "a patient's presence before us in a hospital or office setting becomes for us a moral occasion, a measure of our moral life as it is lived moment to moment." The narratives in this book illustrate this statement. Serious illness is like a storm that pulls at, and sometimes pulls up, the deep roots that are the foundation of identity – self-image, roles, and relationships. It creates tremendous vulnerability, uncertainty, and isolation. Understanding the personal impact of illness leads to the empathy that prompts us, as physicians, to be better educators, to probe a little deeper with a patient who never discusses his personal life, and to ask simple questions such as "How is this illness affecting your life?", "How is your mood?" and "How is your family reacting?" These questions convey the doctor's concern and understanding that the impact of illness is greater than its physical dimensions. They open the door for frank discussions of psychosocial issues with patients, and help us to guide them, as best we can, to maintain or rebuild a life with quality, dignity, and purpose.

> It is a strange but unavoidable quirk in our system that those of us who become doctors are educated and turned loose at a time in our life when personal disease and debility are least likely. I can remember as an intern being frankly surprised at how many people were sick.
>
> . . . This point was dramatized for me recently when I tried to explain it in the course of a lecture to a group of medical students. "We are all patients", I began. "A few of us become physicians as well." I proceeded to develop the argument that we should not think of ourselves as elite, but rather as helpmates to our fellows, whose biology and pathology are, after all, the same as our own. I concluded by urging them to maintain a sense of humility as they pursued their profession, suggesting that this would make them better physicians. This all was said, I reflected later, at precisely the time when they were doing everything in their power to join the medical fraternity. . . . All in all, it was an unpropitious time for the students to receive any message. They were killing themselves trying to

achieve membership in the club while I was telling them the club wasn't all that exclusive.

Fitzhugh Mullan, MD

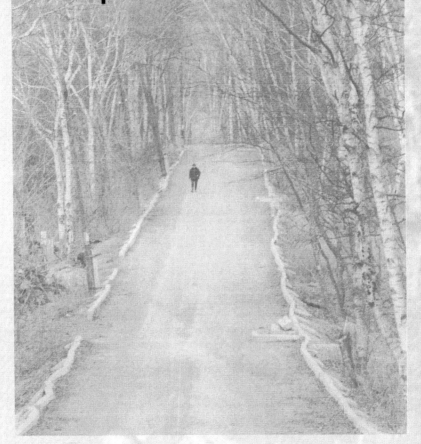

SECTION 1

The Experience of Illness

Illness is the night-side of life, a more onerous citizenship. Everyone who is born holds dual citizenship, in the kingdom of the well and in the kingdom of the sick. Although we prefer to use only the good passport, sooner or later each of us is obliged, at least for a spell, to identify ourselves as citizens of that other place.

Susan Sontag

The Impact of Illness on Identity, Self-Esteem, Roles, and Relationships

Critical illness leaves no aspect of life unchanged. . . . Your relationships, your work, your sense of who you are and who you might become, your sense of what life is and what it ought to be – these all change and the change is terrifying. Twice, as I realized how ill I was, I saw these changes coming and was overwhelmed by them.

Arthur Frank, PhD

At 3 p.m. on otherwise unremarkable October afternoon, I walk into an examination room to meet Mr. Percy, a slightly overweight and out of shape 32-year-old single engineer with sandy brown hair and green eyes. He sits awkwardly in his chair and begins his story, glancing down at notes carefully written on a pad of lined yellow paper.

"It started six months ago, I felt more tired and achy – just thought I was getting old", he says, with a strained laugh, eyes staring down at his hands. ". . . And then this rash – all over my hands and face." He holds out his red chapped-looking hands and then, looking up only briefly to make eye contact, he gestures at his reddened face. As the interview progresses, Mr. Percy talks about his life. He is an introvert with few friends, but he has a very close relationship with his parents. He is an avid golfer and he breeds show dogs.

"I can't keep up when I play golf anymore, and I can't keep up with the dogs. And then, there were these heart palpitations . . ." He pauses. Shifting in his chair, he talks in a quiet and measured tone but, as he tells his story, poor eye contact and an occasional nervous laugh suggest his anxiety and frustration. The dermatologist says that the rash is psoriasis and has started a topical treatment. The cardiologist found nothing but a mild elevation in the creatinine kinase and episodes of benign supraventricular tachicardia – now well controlled with a beta-blocker. However, because of the persistent aching, Mr. Percy's family doctor has sent him for another opinion.

As he talks, a picture starts to form from what initially appear to be random symptoms. The stream of seemingly unconnected events is fitting together into a diagnosis – dermatomyositis. At that moment, with that realization, you find that only part of your mind is listening to the story. The other part, initially excited by solving the puzzle and making the diagnosis, is sobered by the uncomfortable knowledge that the life of the unsuspecting person sitting in front of you is about to change irrevocably.

In the next few months, it becomes clear that Mr. Percy not only has an unusual muscle disease, but is also rapidly losing lung function as a result of obliterative pneumonitis. Within a year, the man sitting in the exam room is not the same person who came for help that day in October – neither physically nor emotionally, neither at work nor at home. He will be 50 pounds heavier, almost bald from medication, and he will need oxygen to carry out the simplest of daily activities. He will be hospitalized multiple times for unexpected complications – a deep venous thrombosis for which he is given an anticoagulant and then a retroperitoneal bleed from his anticoagulation. A Greenfield filter will be placed so that he can be taken off anticoagulation. He will develop diabetes, hypertension, infections, and muscle weakness – all from his corticosteroid treatment. At a follow-up visit, he will reluctantly mention that he has become impotent.

This avid golfer will be too weak to golf, or to work, or to care for his dogs. He will be too embarrassed by his appearance and too limited by his lung disease to socialize with friends. He will depend increasingly on his parents for help – to make meals, clean his house, keep him company – and for financial support. The quiet, organized man with an ironic sense of humor will be replaced by an anxious, often tearful, and increasingly angry and bitter person, in rumpled clothing covered with dog hair. His identity – that complex composite made up of his appearance, interests, talents, attributes, relationships, and roles – will change.

IDENTITY

As it did for Mr. Percy, serious illness can affect every aspect of identity. Dr. Eric Cassel wrote:

> A person has roles. I am a husband, a father, a physician, a teacher, a brother, an orphaned son, and an uncle. People are their roles and each role has rules. Together, the rules that guide the performance of the roles make up a complex set of entitlements and limitations of responsibility and privilege. By middle age, the roles may be so firmly set that disease can lead to the virtual destruction of a person by making the performance of his or her roles impossible. Whether the patient is a doctor who cannot doctor or a mother who cannot mother, he or she is diminished by the loss of function.

Arthur Frank, a medical sociologist, described the effect of his cancer on his identity as follows:

> Disease changed my life as husband, father, professor, and everything else. I had learned to be dependent. I was unreliable in practical matters and often in emotional ones as well, and incapable of doing tasks that I had considered normal. It was no small thing to rediscover myself as I changed.
>
> *Arthur Frank, PhD*

PERSONAL APPEARANCE, SELF-IMAGE, AND SELF-ESTEEM

Illnesses that change your appearance can have a demoralizing impact on self-image and self-esteem. Whether it is weight loss or weight gain (related to medicines or inactivity), loss of muscle strength and stamina, hair loss, or changes in complexion such as rashes or acne, the physical impact of illness can make you feel as if you are losing the person you used to be. Surgical procedures such as mastectomy, colostomies, and amputations are an abrupt assault on the body, and change physical identity.

What is even more frustrating for patients is that physicians often do not fully prepare them for the physical changes that come with serious illness and treatment. Although he had been warned about weight gain and diabetes, Mr. Percy was surprised and worried when he developed acne, increased hair growth on his face and body, insomnia and mood swings, and later cataracts from his corticosteroid treatment. Frequent, unexpected, and not under his control, these complications and the physical and emotional changes that they caused left him feeling helpless and anxious. Patients must watch, wait, and worry. The experience is demoralizing.

The following excerpts from memoirs of and interviews with patients capture the profound impact of illness on appearance, self-image, and self-esteem.

Hair loss from chemotherapy

. . . To be completely bald at my age was a bit unusual but was not in itself stigmatizing. I had never thought of hair loss itself as one of life's great problems. But losing my hair all at once was traumatic, even if my age and gender reduced the trauma.

Arthur Frank, PhD

Loss of muscle tone in the abdomen from a spinal cord tumor

An even more visible mark stared at me one morning as I staggered into Marcia and Paul's big bathroom and glimpsed my naked waist in the mirror. Overnight, my gut had collapsed. My waist was at least 10 inches bigger than it had been the previous night. In those few hours, with no prior weakness, I'd lost all power to contract my guts and I never got it back. . . . I had been a fairly presentable man; this was my first big loss of ground in the department of personal pride . . .

Reynolds Price

Body changes due to glucocorticoid use

Throughout those weeks I was on high doses of the steroid . . . and the drug's notorious external signs soon began to appear, the mutilations of Cushing syndrome. They included a swollen and sodden moon face, the start of a buffalo hump of fat on the upper back, a roaring appetite for food, and – worst – exhausting and unpredictable swings of mood.

. . . I was still unable to write.

Reynolds Price

Changes in thinking and emotional responses due to glucocorticoid treatment

After discharge on 60 mg of prednisone and 2 g of Azulfidine, I did well for about two weeks. Then I began to have problems concentrating and memorizing. Soon, I realized that I didn't understand what I was reading. Thinking was difficult and I was restless all the time. Eventually, I became so disorganized that I had to drop all my courses. Over the next two weeks, things became worse. I couldn't even read the newspaper headlines – the words made no sense. I enjoyed nothing and could not imagine anything that could make me happy again. . . . when I was awake, I would cry or eat ravenously. The smallest task demanded great effort, and when I thought about killing myself, it loomed like an insurmountable mission.

Louise Scott, MD

Physical effects of many surgeries and radiation

My physical limitation created the sensation of a strangely accelerated aging process that left my shell looking 33 years old while turning my insides into those of an octogenarian. I hoped that there was more to come in the way of regained strength and endurance, but I was sure that my permanent clout was diminished. . . . The incremental demands of age, the steady pickpocketing that happens to us all, seemed like nothing compared to the Brink's robbery that had been performed on my body.

Fitzhugh Mullan, MD

Changes in bowel function with ulcerative colitis

As my functioning became compromised in this way, I began to hate my body. I joked about trade-offs, but beneath the levity was an increasing shame, guilt, and dislike for myself. I felt betrayed. It was as if my body had suddenly and unpredictably turned on me; my most trusted friend had turned into my biggest adversary. I felt dirty, smelly, and unfeminine. My self-esteem, so inextricably linked to an integral image of myself, eroded further.

Judith Alexander Brice, MD

John Updike writing of his psoriasis

> Psoriasis keeps you thinking. Strategies of concealment ramify, and self-examination is endless. You are forced to the mirror, again and again, psoriasis compels narcissism, if we can suppose a Narcissus who does not like what he saw. In certain lights, your face looks passable, in slightly different other lights, not. Shaving mirrors and rearview mirrors in automobiles are merciless, whereas smoky mirrors in airplane bathrooms are especially flattering and soothing: one's face looks as tawny as a movie star's. . . . I cannot pass a reflecting surface on the street without glancing in, in hopes that I have somehow changed. . . . One hates one's abnormal, erupting skin but is led into brooding, solicitous attention toward it.

ROLES AT HOME

When you ask how the couple are doing, the man shakes his head and says "I will be happy if I never see another one of those frozen casseroles dropped off by some mother at the school again." They do not make eye contact.

It's just an offhand comment, but it is a statement that suggests the slow breakdown of a marriage. Maryanne Stokes, a 32-year-old mother of 5-year-old twin girls, is sitting in the office with her husband. She is well dressed, her hair and make-up perfectly done, and she looks well. Her husband, a businessman who believes in self-discipline, hard work, and exercise, is sitting beside her. Maryanne was diagnosed with multiple sclerosis (MS) two years ago. After a year of relative stability, she was admitted for an unanticipated exacerbation of her MS that left her bedridden, but now she is able to walk again with a cane. Just 2 weeks after discharge from the rehabilitation unit, she has come in for a follow-up appointment, and although on the surface they both look fine, the comment is a clue that things are not going well. During the visit, it becomes clear that Mrs. Stokes has become more passive and depressed in response to her setbacks. Her husband has taken over the management of her medical care, but seems to be doing it more out of duty and obligation than affection.

Mrs. Stokes comes by herself for the next few visits. When you ask how she is coping, she admits that she feels she is playing a role as mother and wife. She can no longer attend the children's after-school activities, clean the house, cook the meals or socialize with the other mothers through clubs and activities at school. She is no longer one of them – she is the outsider who needs help. Just driving the car to pick up the children is difficult, and she needs almost full-time help at home. She suspects that her husband thinks she could do more if she really tried. The cost of her medical care, the help at home, and her depression have had a significant impact on her relationship with her husband, and she feels now that she has a marriage in name only. She is lonely, dispirited, and depressed. The only people from whom she receives unconditional love and support are her parents and siblings, who live out of state. The only goal that motivates her is to care for and preserve her relationship with her children.

Illnesses like this – those that cause significant changes in energy, mood, physical function, and endurance – affect a parent's ability to function at home, and can cause profound changes in roles within the family. It may be more difficult to be the caretaker, to make the meals, to drive the children to activities, to keep the household going, to play and coach sports with friends and children, to attend games, and to enjoy the hobbies around which you have built relationships. Medical appointments prevent parents from reliably being at home when their children return from school, and fatigue and pain can make it difficult to listen, to make snacks, and to help with homework even if they are home. The consequences of living on a more limited income can be demoralizing for the breadwinners.

Those who are lucky will find friends and family to help with these activities. However, even this help comes at a cost. The person who is ill can feel isolated, left out of the family's routine, guilty about their inability to perform essential roles in the family and about imposing on others for help, and jealous or resentful of the partner or friends who take over their roles. Relying on others to care for their children and listen to their children's problems often leaves a parent out of the important relationships that previously brought them joy and a feeling of accomplishment.

Fitzhugh Mullan wrote about his isolation from his family during prolonged hospitalization and treatment for cancer and the complications associated with that treatment:

> In the early days of my illness . . . Meghan and Judy spent a tremendous amount of time together and embarked on numerous projects of which I was not a part. . . . While I understood that Judy was protecting my energies by doing more than her share of the child rearing . . . I felt left out sometimes. I couldn't object since I had no alternative, but at intervals I felt envious – and even jealous – of the intimacy they shared in many areas.

For many, the support of friends and family can be surprisingly short-lived in a chronic illness, especially if there are no visible signs of illness and the symptoms are mostly "constitutional", such as fatigue, weakness, pain, anxiety, or depression. After a few months, as the other stresses of day-to-day life crowd back in, children usually return to their naturally self-absorbed lives, tired partners voice their frustrations about the dishes and the laundry or the work around the house that are not done or the decrease in the family's income, and family and friends become tired of hearing about the illness, but those who are seriously ill may have little else to talk about, and silence ensues.

ROLES AT WORK

While he was unable to work, Mr. Percy was amazed to find that he missed his job and his co-workers – a job that he previously considered boring. Being home alone but unable to get out and do things, without any routine, increased his anxiety and isolation. For most people, roles at work (even at a job they dislike), relationships with the people with whom they work, and the recognition that they receive for what they do are integral parts of their identity. Loss of a work identity, of the rewards that come from doing a job well, of the social interactions, and of outside validation of skills and contributions leads to significant loss of self-esteem. The financial stress of disability adds to vulnerability, guilt, and lack of control over life.

Even if return to work is possible, the transition is likely to be difficult. Physical factors such as fatigue, pain, and weakness, and physical disabilities, as well as psychological factors such as anxiety, anger, and depression affect performance. Many people notice changes in their thinking and find that they can no longer concentrate, read, problem solve, or organize their working day. The author and poet, Reynolds Price, found that he was unable to write for months after he became paralyzed as a result of a spinal cord tumor:

> As in all hospitals, time bore down between events. For me it hung surprisingly heavy, because for the first time since grade school, I'd run head on into a block on my work. . . . Stranger still, I found myself unable to read anything longer than a magazine article. My eyes were normal but my patience was gone . . .
>
> *Reynolds Price*

And then there is the difficult decision about how much information to give to employers and colleagues. Although most people want the help and support of colleagues at work during and after an illness, many worry about the loss of privacy and the possible threat to their job security. Due to feeling awkward about discussing illness or unsure of what to say, co-workers may avoid contact or meaningful discussions. Those who don't understand the impact of illness frequently do not offer appropriate support. The lack of support from colleagues and employers can cause disappointment, anger, resentment, and isolation.

Even if they are initially helpful, co-workers and employers often don't understand the long-term aspects of illness, and may have inappropriate expectations about the person's ability to return to their normal work roles and responsibilities. Arthur Frank describes a typical experience. During his treatment for cancer, he initially felt supported by colleagues and the university where he worked. However, that support dwindled as he tried to return to the demands of an academic position:

> While I was in active treatment, the university where I worked was most solicitous. . . . But as soon as treatment ended, the other institutional face appeared. Some of the same people now asked for the work that I was supposed to be doing. It didn't count that I had been ill; in the annual assessment written about each faculty member, the time of my illness was described as showing a "lack of scholarly productivity." I had to remind the administrator who wrote the report to specify that this lack was due to illness. But illness does not matter for institutions, any more than pregnancy matters or caring for someone else who is ill matters. . . . Gaps in résumés are institutional stigmas. Since most of us have to work, it is hard for ill persons to resist accepting productivity as the measure of our worth.
>
> *Arthur Frank, PhD*

Paradoxically, employers or supervisors may be unwilling to give an employee who has recovered from a serious illness a position with the same responsibilities and authority. Long after recovery, they are frequently not offered promotions and opportunities for advancement because of the employer's unwillingness to "take a risk" – putting the interests of the organization first. Some people find that their job disappears during their illness.

Drs. Mandell and Spiro wrote about the experience of an academic physician who was diagnosed with melanoma:

There is a practical reason why physicians so rarely write about getting sick. Practicing physicians usually need to maintain an aura of perfection, for the doctor who talks about being sick may lose his practice. Reliability and availability are key. The powerful chairman of an internal medicine department knew that having melanoma took away his future: he could not be counted on to be there. "My previous inborn sense of immortality [was] totally destroyed. . . . The school leaders . . . also discounted my future. . . . I had no future and the present was in disarray, and even my professional past, which was the background of the work I was doing and was about to do more of, was made to look wasted."

When Doctors Get Sick

> Illness excuses people from their normal responsibilities, but the cost of being excused is greater than it appears at first. An excuse is also an exclusion.
>
> ARTHUR FRANK, PHD

RELATIONSHIPS

Serious illness can distance you from personal and physical relationships. It can set you apart from something as simple as a touch or a hug from friends and family, as well as more complex personal and sexual relationships. People may be less likely to make physical contact because of their fear that they will cause pain, because they find the person less attractive, or because they are unsure if it is appropriate. Those who are ill sometimes withdraw, both physically and psychologically. They may be embarrassed by their appearance or too fatigued, anxious, or depressed to participate in social and sexual relationships.

After treatment for cancer and multiple surgeries and complications, Fitzhugh Mullan wrote:

> There is simply nothing sexy about vomiting, weight loss, surgery, or scars. I remember wondering . . . if Judy would still find me attractive after all that had been done to me. After weeks of treatment and for many months afterwards I hardly cared, since I felt so physically wretched. In fact, for a long period I felt completely asexual. In much the same way that I lost track of my identity as a physician during my initial long hospitalization, I gradually became oblivious to my identity as a man. . . . I didn't feel

romantic, I didn't act romantic, and I wasn't treated romantically.

Recovery meant once again becoming something other than a neuter. I had to find out first of all if my body would function after months of surgery, chemotherapy, radiation, and physical wastage.

Reynolds Price also described a loss of sexual desire during and after treatment for spinal cord cancer that left him paralyzed:

> I also hoped in those hospital days, although a lot less strongly than I'd have guessed, that sexual desire would soon revive and reach outside me. . . . But from the moment I'd waked after surgery, the hunger to know and please other bodies was suddenly and inexplicably gone for the first time in nearly 40 years.

Serious illness can be stigmatizing, causing exclusion and embarrassment, especially if it is associated with significant physical or mental disability or disfigurement. Dr. Kay Redfield Jamison, a faculty member at Johns Hopkins School of Medicine, wrote about the stigma of her diagnosis of bipolar illness and the difficulty she had discussing it with friends and colleagues:

> There is no easy way to tell other people that you have manic-depressive illness; if there is, I haven't found it. So despite the fact that most people I have told have been very understanding – some remarkably so – I remain haunted by those occasions when the response was unkind, condescending, or lacking in even a semblance of empathy. . . . Too, I have been very concerned, perhaps unduly so, with how knowing that I have manic-depressive illness will affect people's perception of who
> I am and what I do.

When people become seriously ill they often feel isolated, set apart from their closest friends and family, and forced to unwillingly join a small group of vulnerable outsiders. They notice, usually for the first time, that the

> Illness can crowd out talk.
>
> ARTHUR FRANK, PHD

world is divided into two groups – those who have their health, are in control of their lives, and are moving forward, and those who are not. Their day-to-day activities and concerns change. While friends, family, and associates are talking about the weekend ball game, vacation plans, work, and social events, they are living a more physically limited life, much of which is taken up by medical treatment. The future is uncertain and they are often unable to participate in the activities and interests that previously connected them to friends, family, and the world in general. Because much of their time, energy, and thoughts are focused on "getting back" to being the healthy person they used to be, dealing with the illness can dominate their life.

Arthur Frank described his isolation during his treatment for cancer. The cancer diagnosis was a stigma that he did not want to discuss with his friends, so he withdrew from social situations:

> Whenever I told someone that I had cancer I felt myself tighten as I said it. Saying the word "cancer", my whole body began to defend itself. This did not happen when I told people I was having a heart problem. A heart attack was simply bad news. But I never stopped thinking that cancer said something about my worth as a person. The difference between heart attack and cancer is stigma. . . . During my active treatment I never found a way of dealing with my sense of stigma.

> . . . Heart attacks are invisible on the body's surface. To myself and others, I looked no different. One wears cancer. My own visible stigmas were hair loss and my intravenous line. . . . The sad answer is that I experienced the visible signs of cancer as defects not just in my appearance but in myself.

> . . . But I did not want to believe I had cancer, and others did not want to hear about that possibility. My awkward attempts to avoid commitments I was not sure I could fulfill only made people think I was distancing myself from them. I acted not from lack of friendship but because my body was taking me out of the natural flow of plans and expectations. Others took planning for granted; my future was pervaded by uncertainty. I lost my sense of belonging.

But at home, as in the hospital, the ill person is eventually alone with illness.

———————————

ARTHUR FRANK, PHD

The awkwardness of friends, family, and co-workers who don't know what to say or how to respond increases isolation. Some people will avoid friends or family members during serious illness, and others will not talk about the illness because they are worried that conversation might lead to an emotion – anger, sadness, depression, or defensiveness – that will make them or the person who is ill uncomfortable.

Hospitalization compounds isolation – taking you into a sterile world and away from friends, family, your daily routine, and a familiar environment over which you have some control. Dr. Eric Cassel wrote about serious illness as follows:

> The world around the sick person shrinks to such a small space, scarcely larger than his own body – the box of tissues on the bed, the bed itself, and perhaps the room. Someone may be nearby but seems not to be there, so faint is the connection with others. The patient becomes disconnected from the world, feeling as though it would be fearfully easy to fall off. So pervasive is the helplessness that distress, pain, and weakness may appear to be the only realities. Understanding fails and sustained thought seems difficult to achieve. All control of the world is gone. . . . The patient is dependent on all around him. . . . As illness deepens, connections are increasingly cut off . . .

Comfort and consolation are often best found in relationships with other people who have been ill. In their company, and because of the shared experience, the person who is seriously ill can relax and exchange stories without feeling guilty or that they are a burden. These relationships provide a place in which to share strategies about how to live and cope with illness, laugh about the absurdities and indignities encountered during their medical care, and offer each other advice, consolation, and hope. Arthur Frank described it like this:

> Those who best affirmed my experience were often people who had been through critical illness themselves or with someone close. We did not necessarily talk a great deal about specific experiences, but these friends seemed to be able to look at me clearly and

I was feeling lonely and isolated. I had no friends or peers who were severely ill or who had cancer.

FITZHUGH MULLAN, MD

to accept what they saw. They rarely tried to cheer me up, but being with them did cheer me up. Human suffering becomes bearable when we share it. When we know that someone recognizes our pain we can let go of it. The power of recognition to reduce suffering cannot be explained, but it seems fundamental to our humanity.

Emotional Responses to Serious Illness

How the individual handles being sick reflects his attitudes, defenses, strengths, weaknesses and philosophy of life.

Drs. Reiser and Rosen

Jean Reed is 69 years old and recently widowed. Her husband died of lymphoma a few months ago. A pale, small, anxious woman with a pleasant wrinkled face and only wisps of gray hair left on her head, Jean has significant deformity of most of her joints due to rheumatoid arthritis. I have known Jean for years. Originally from the Aran Islands, she answers all my questions with a thoughtful and direct look and responds, "Well, you know doctor . . ." as she launches into a discussion with her lyrical accent. She was diagnosed in her twenties when there were no effective treatments for arthritis, and she has had multiple complications – severe joint deformities and multiple replacements, paper-thin skin, and osteoporosis and fractures. She has little use of her hands and has been completely dependent on her husband for decades.

At each visit, she nervously reviews every symptom and every medical problem that has occurred since she was last seen. Before she goes, she makes sure that I have received every outside lab test, and she frequently calls back with questions she forgot to ask during the visit – sometimes from the waiting room as she leaves.

I took care of Jean for years before she told me about her husband's multiple affairs. The subject came up one day after she arrived, more anxious and agitated than usual, for her regular office visit. She complained about her husband's plans to buy a convertible. Because of her severe osteoporosis, she was worried that the car wouldn't offer her enough protection from fractures if they were in an accident. As she started to cry, she said, "Well, you know doctor . . ." and then related the long story of her husband's multiple relationships and open flirtations with other women at social gatherings. As she talked, I remembered that over the years, as they sat together during office visits, I had found myself wondering how her husband had coped with the changes in his life that Jean's illness had brought. I could easily imagine them as a young, attractive couple just married and full of optimism and plans for the future, but I had more difficulty understanding how their life, their expectations, their view of themselves and each other, and their relationship must have gradually changed and how ill equipped they probably were to deal with this.

"My daughters know", she said, almost matter of factly. "But there is really nothing I can do. I would love to go back to my family home and I know my cousins would help to care for me, but I can't get these expensive medications there."

Jean's disease and its complications leave her completely vulnerable and dependent. For most of her life, she lived with an illness for which there were no effective treatments and over which she had little control. Years later, when her disease stabilized on new treatment, she was perpetually waiting for the "other shoe to drop." After a fruitless year-long work-up for weight loss, which her family doctor and I finally agreed was most likely due to depression, she refused prescriptions for antidepressants.

Three years before his death, Jean's husband, an avid golfer, skier, and athlete, was diagnosed with lymphoma. In the years that followed, he and Jean were reconciled. As he went from doctor to doctor, receiving chemotherapy and radiation treatments, she was there at his side doing the only thing she could still physically do – keep him company and give him advice. He had joined the club to which Jean was a lifetime member, and they were finally able to support one another.

I didn't see Jean for months after her husband's death. I had heard that a niece from Canada had come to live with the couple before he died, and then stayed on until Jean could make some decisions about what to do next. When she arrived at the office 6 months later, I was surprised to see that she had gained weight – about 10 pounds – and that she was laughing and chatting in an animated way with her niece. She was not the anxious, sad woman I had seen over so many visits. When I remarked about her weight gain, she gestured to her niece, a young, attractive woman sitting beside her, and said laughing, "Well, you know doctor, Nancy is a gourmet cook and she is fattening me up!" This new relationship provided the care and security that Jean needed to go on with life.

VULNERABILITY, UNCERTAINTY, AND LOSS OF CONTROL

Jean had to deal with the three most difficult challenges of serious illness – vulnerability, uncertainty, and lack of control. This triad is at the root of many of the emotional responses to illness. People worry that everything important in life – physical independence, relationships with children, spouse, and friends, their career, and perhaps life itself – could be lost or changed. The future is uncertain and the stakes are high. Because of relapses, exacerbations, and complications of illness and treatment, the body can't be relied upon to function reliably. You don't know whether the life that you have lived will continue and, if it does, whether it will ever be the same again. And, like Jean, you may have little control over the course or outcome.

Fear is the natural human response to this dilemma. Dr. Mary O'Flaherty Horn, an internist, wrote about the fear that she felt when she was diagnosed with amyotrophic lateral sclerosis (ALS):

> I had certainly been in large medical centers before; therefore, there was no reason to feel overwhelmed. I myself am a well-trained internist from a large university – I knew the scene – but this summer morning was different. I was tired and scared. Just two weeks before I had been told that the slurred speech that had been progressing for several months was probably caused by amyotrophic lateral sclerosis (ALS). They'd said 2 to 5 years and, as a physician, I knew all too well the grim prognosis and disheartening lack of therapy associated with my diagnosis.

All aspects of routine medical care lead to a loss of control over time. There are hours of waiting – waiting in offices to be seen or waiting on the telephone to make contact with medical professionals to discuss a problem, obtain test results, make appointments or get referrals. You spend long hours on the telephone to insurance companies and billing offices as you try to sort out confusing medical bills. If the doctor is late, the line at the lab is long, or the tests results have not come back, you must wait, call again, or cajole the person at the end of the phone to find someone who can help you. Lack of control over the schedule of tests and treatment can disrupt the transition back to work and the ability to reliably meet schedules at home. Patients often feel that their time has no value.

Hospitalization increases vulnerability. For patients, the hospital is a foreign place with acrid unpleasant odors that lacks sunlight, fresh air, and the familiar and reassuring comforts of home. People experience a loss of privacy and control over medical decisions and the systems and people who deliver care. Other people control the tests, the treatments, the schedule, and the decisions. Patients are expected to be passive participants, and those who try to have more control over the process often find themselves in a power struggle with everyone from the receptionist, transport personnel, and lab technicians to the nurses and doctors – all of whom are resistant to their input.

Dr. Judith Alexander Brice wrote about her experience of loss of control while she was hospitalized for a flare-up of Crohn's disease:

> During these hospitalizations . . . I found it very difficult to switch gears. As a doctor, I was functioning in a profession of strength, of intellectual activity, of control, and of independence. These qualities did not easily mesh with that of a passive, compliant patient. One minute I was the psychiatric consultant heading up case conferences, seeing private patients, and supervising residents. In my personal life I was running the routine of a household, relating to the needs of my husband, and taking care of a 2-year-old son. The next moment I was in the hospital, with everyone from the maintenance crew and the janitorial staff to the medical staff feeling entitled to enter my room without knocking. Within hours of being in charge of my life, I suddenly found myself surrendering control over almost every aspect of my daily routine. Social boundaries, professional boundaries, personal boundaries were repeatedly subject to thoughtless violation. Doctors walked into the bathroom to examine me on the commode. Well-intentioned and unthinking volunteer staff walked into my room unannounced and interrupted my very personal conversations to deliver my mail. Maintenance staff were there to greet me when I walked out of the shower. Nursing staff entered my room at night, clanging ice pitchers and laying out new linen. I didn't want clean pajamas; I was a light sleeper and wanted rest. I wanted a modicum of privacy, respect, and control.

During the second hospitalization in March of 1982, I felt as if I found the answer. I put a sign on the door requesting politely that people knock and wait for an answer before entering. I am convinced that this wish for a normal modicum of privacy branded me as a kook among the nursing staff. I was to pay dearly for it during my subsequent hospitalization. The routine, I found out, was bigger than I.

In the following excerpt, Reynolds Price describes his feeling about hospitalization on the drive from his familiar and safe home in the woods of North Carolina back to the hospital:

> . . . as we drove away from the house again in the late afternoon, I couldn't help trying to burn certain sights deep into my brain – the old beech trees with trunks the color and shape of elephant legs, the pond that for so many years had harbored a particular blue heron, the house itself that had sheltered me and my friends for nineteen years. . . . Whatever the intangible fears I was fleeing, when it came to thinking about [the] hospital, I knew precisely what I was fleeing – an actual building and a very few members of its staff who in my mind (for right or wrong) now meant only pain and death.

A patient told me a story that helped me to understand the imbalance of power and control in medical care. Mrs. Brown is a bright, insightful, and attractive 40-year-old mother of three from a prominent local family. Two years ago, she developed unexplained fatigue and, after a trip to the local ER and hospitalization, she was told that she had irreversible kidney failure. With determination, she weathered a year of dialysis, exercising regularly, rushing home after each dialysis treatment to meet her children from the bus, supported by the anticipation of a transplant. A year later, after the transplanted kidney was rejected, she was back on dialysis but, with the same resolve, she was working towards a second transplant.

When I saw her in the office that day, she was two years into the illness and obviously exhausted by infections, hospitalizations, and setbacks. She had given up on her exercise program and was struggling to stay out of bed from the time her children came home from school to the time they went to bed at night. At the end of the visit, I gave her a lab order to bring to the dialysis unit for blood tests to be done the following day. "Oh no", she smiled nervously, "I can't do that." When I looked confused, she said, "I don't want to ask for anything special. The nurses decide what order we start dialysis. Some people are in no rush – they socialize and chat during dialysis. But I have to get home for the bus. If you ask for anything special or they think you are demanding, they put you on last." Her education, good looks, and upper-middle-class status did not protect her. She was vulnerable, she needed their help, and she had to play by their rules.

FEAR AND ANXIETY

As time goes on, intense feelings of fear often transform into low-grade, chronic anxiety that patients like Jean Reed show us every day. This anxiety usually lasts for years, even into recovery. It becomes the free-floating worry that the body can no longer be trusted, that something could go wrong at any time. Fitzhugh Mullan, an academic internist who was diagnosed with seminoma early in his career, described the fear and anxiety that his treatment for cancer and its complications and frequent setbacks caused:

> It was strange to regard my body with suspicion. . . . I had never given much thought to the functioning or malfunctioning of my body's various parts. I assumed that they would do pretty good and they did. The cancer in my chest destroyed all of that, absolutely and permanently. No longer was I confident in my body. It had failed me.
>
> . . . Friends in the hospital congratulated me on my impending departure. I had made it through therapy and, after 2 months, was going home, where things would be better. I didn't feel that way about it at all. I had arrived in the hospital seemingly healthy, mentally intact, and ready to do battle. Now I was leaving the hospital in a wheelchair, emaciated, unable to swallow, troubled by breathing, and acutely depressed. . . . On my last morning of radiation therapy before I was to leave the hospital, I suffered an incredible spasm of anxiety. Crying did no good. Vomiting, spitting, and belching were in no way cathartic. There seemed to be no avenue of escape from the constant fear and nausea that I felt. . . . I had no idea of what was happening that day except that my life, or what was left of it, was coming to a head. In spite of my abhorrence of the hospital, I feared leaving it. . . . Deep within me I could not accept being cut adrift to fend for myself. I had become a slave of my therapies.

In life-threatening illnesses, a person's relationship with their body is altered so dramatically that they may never completely forget the profound emotional impact of illness. Drs. Reiser and Rosen wrote, "Of course, the terror recedes and the defenses return, but at some level a person who has been seriously ill has seen his own mortality. Such a person has been altered – wiser on occasion, often not – but not the same."

Repeated setbacks and complications also contribute to anxiety – the worry that, without notice or warning, anything could go wrong at any time and the consequences could be dire. To deal with this vulnerability, patients often spend more and more time analyzing symptoms in an attempt to ward off impending disaster. Like Jean Reed, people with chronic illness often dwell on bodily symptoms and the small details of how they feel, looking for clues that will allow them to ward off the next complication and give them some control. Arthur Kleinman wrote, "Attention is vigorously focused, sometimes hour by hour, to the specifics of circumstances and events that could be potential sources of worsening. There is a daily quest for control of the known provoking agents. The chronically ill become interpreters of good and bad omens. They are archivists searching a disorganized file of past experiences."

> . . . I can see in the meticulous entries that I rapidly developed an obsessive fascination with my body and its momentary symptoms.
>
> **REYNOLDS PRICE**

In the following excerpt, Fitzhugh Mullan discusses his obsessive attention to bodily symptoms caused by his overwhelming anxiety that the cancer would recur:

> A new problem began to emerge at this point: I began to be obsessed by the question of whether the tumor would reappear. . . . And so, fearfully, humorlessly, I began to study my body wondering where they might show up. . . . I couldn't shave without finding a distended blood vessel or sleep without suffering a "night sweat." I attached a morbid diagnosis to every lump or rash I could discover. . . . The gnawing, self-consumptive fear of recurrence is a constant and destructive phenomenon.

. . . Little things would often trip me up. One evening in a beautiful setting at an open-air concert . . . I coughed and felt a new pain in my chest. The concert was over for me. The music, the people, the setting all faded into the background as I wrestled with a terrible onrush of anxiety. The pain, like so many others, faded out with time. . . . I thought about what a terrible and inaccurate gauge of the body the mind can be. Frequently, after a period of well-being, I would wake in the morning feeling ill. . . . Ill most often meant feeling pokey, subpar, a little nauseated, or just a little flimsy. If anxiety wasn't part of the symptomatology, it certainly added itself to the brew. . . . Occasionally the onset of an intercurrent illness was indeed the culprit. A fellow cancer patient described it as the "Goody-it's-the-flu-syndrome" . . . the relief of being able to put a name and a good prognosis on a set of vague symptoms is a joy I came to appreciate.

The complications and setback of severe illness force people to live at the margins where even small changes in health can be irretrievable and lead to a loss of independence. Arthur Kleinman describes the impact of vulnerability as follows:

The undercurrent of chronic illness is like a volcano: it does not go away. It menaces. It erupts. It is out of control. One damned thing follows another. Confronting crisis is only part of the total picture. The rest is coming to grips with the mundaneness of worries over whether one can negotiate a curb . . . make it to the bathroom quickly enough, eat breakfast without vomiting . . . sleep through the night, attempt sexual intercourse, make plans for a trip . . . or just plain face up to the myriad of difficulties that make life feel burdened, uncomfortable, and all too often desperate.

Serious illness can make people feel physically and emotionally "locked in." Physical symptoms such as pain and nausea, and emotional symptoms such as anxiety and depression make it difficult to focus on or care for others or attend to the surrounding world. The quest to stay well and therefore to stay "safe" leads to a state of almost unavoidable self-absorption. Dwelling on the meaning of physical symptoms often causes people to neglect their relationships with friends, family, and children, and makes it difficult to see the joy in day-to-day life. Reluctance or inability to participate in social activities leads to further isolation and low self-esteem, and strains relationships.

GUILT, ANGER, AND MOURNING

Inevitably, the diagnosis of serious illness raises the question "Why me?" It is difficult to find consolation for the grief that comes when you lose the life you expected to live. Especially if you think, correctly or incorrectly, that it was preventable. Many people are convinced that they are personally responsible for their illness – through what they either have or haven't done: "I let myself get too stressed", "I didn't see the warning signs", "I should have eaten better, exercised more, come in sooner for a check-up."

Parents can feel overwhelming guilt about the impact of their illness on their children. Jennifer Brown's greatest concern and regret was the impact of repeated and often unexpected hospitalizations on her children. Dr. Judith Alexander Brice was hospitalized emergently for surgery for an ileostomy. She wrote about her feelings when she had to leave her son for hospitalizations:

> My guilt and despair surfaced in an unimaginable intensity. I had felt incredibly saddened each time I'd had to leave my son and go into the hospital. I was devoted to him, and I knew he could not comprehend what was happening. I felt tremendously sad that he was having to go through this immense upheaval. Unfortunately, my emotional conviction that if I'd been smarter I could have avoided this mess resulted in my feeling overwhelmed by guilt. Cognitively I knew it was not true. Emotionally, however, I felt that it was my fault that my son was having to endure such pain and emotional trauma at such a young age. I was mercilessly hard on myself . . .

Patients often look back at the decisions that they or their physicians made, complications that occurred, and delays in diagnosis and wonder "What if . . .? Would things have been different?" Many people are paralyzed by anger about their loss of health and independence, frustrated by a healthcare system and insurance programs that are not organized to be responsive to their needs, and disappointed with friends and colleagues who do not offer appropriate support or who disappear altogether. Fitzhugh Mullan experienced multiple setbacks during his cancer treatment, including wound and bone infections that required repeated surgeries. He wrote:

> I think repeatedly about the operations I have undergone – particularly the first one. I wonder what if the biopsy had gone well and there had been no bleeding and no thoracotomy? What if, what if . . .? Like a Monday morning

quarterback, I run and rerun the plays in my mind fretting over a dropped pass and a missed block. During the hospitalization to rebuild my chest, particularly, I spent endless frustrated hours wallowing in these thoughts. But, even now, at this distance, the possibilities that things might have gone better and the results might have been more benign has an allure that I cannot avoid. This is especially preoccupying when I am feeling sorry for myself for one reason or another.

. . . In the weeks that followed I was to weep frequently and suddenly without immediate cause. The disease and its treatment so stripped me of my defenses that any event with the least bit of emotional content caused me to cry. I cried over television news stories . . . as well as the many kind letters I received from friends. Talking with Judy about our future was always interrupted with a tearful episode or two on my part. While the tears were honest and cathartic, they were also an annoying impediment to almost any serious conversation. In retrospect, I suppose they were tears of impotence and anger, tears of a spirit that had been blindsided by disease. As the weeks passed, my raw emotions became rawer and my sense of self-pity deepened.

DEPRESSION

A life of dealing with the losses that illness and setbacks impose can lead to depression and burnout, and to giving up. In his book, *The Illness Narratives*, Arthur Kleinman describes a hospitalized woman whom he was asked to see for depression. She had severe diabetes, but she had been able to maintain a positive, "take-charge" attitude. She cared for her family, kept all her appointments, followed a strict diet, and complied with all of her medication prescriptions. At first, she managed setbacks and hospitalizations with optimism and persistence. Eventually, however, vascular disease led to heart failure that significantly limited her activity and affected her ability to care for her family. Finally, after multiple hospitalizations for foot infections, an amputation was recommended by her physicians. Dr. Kleinman wrote:

As the mundane discomforts accumulate, they take over everyday life. They become all an ill person has to look forward to. And one day, after many days with nothing to look forward to, that person changes. She doesn't decide to change or even perceive that she has changed, but she has. She has been worn away and she doesn't care anymore. Among caregivers, this change is referred to as burnout.

The environment in which we provide care is often demoralizing. Reynolds Price described the depressing atmosphere of the radiation therapy clinics:

> Admittedly the visible surroundings of the clinic were hardly encouraging. Despite alert nurses and plates of cookies, the upbeat ochre-colored walls, and the astrological secretary, nothing could muffle the forbidden sight of the men and women in the small waiting room. Their varying states of emaciation and the look of their skin – blue, ashen, or jaundiced – were only heightened by our efforts at whispering mutual cheer among us. We tended to offer each other box scores – "I've only got six treatments to go, then I am done for life. How about you?"

After multiple setbacks and complications, Fitzhugh Mullan felt overwhelmed by his illness and wrote:

> I only know that during this time I felt blighted physically and overrun psychologically. I am sure that deep within me I was furious with the fates that had brought me to my knees in youth. . . . I was past being angry. What I do remember feeling was despair. My glass, it seemed to me now, was truly half empty. Why had I been singled out to receive this blow? Why would I not be able to see my grandchildren or realize my full skills as a physician? Why would my parents have to see me, their oldest son, die? Why did I have to vomit and tremble? Why did my hair have to come out by the combful? Why? Why? Why? . . . Guilt was also a theme in the search for the reason for my cancer.

Burnout, or giving up, is more likely to occur when patients experience multiple complications and setbacks over which, despite their best efforts, they have no control. Eventually they give up – especially if they are fatigued, physically weak, or have exhausted their personal and financial support.

People who have had little control in their personal life, due to their social environment, financial limitations, or lack of education, often approach illness more passively from the start, and are less likely to be hopeful that anything they do in terms of treatment will affect the outcome.

Coping and Renewal

If recovery is to be taken as the ideal, how is it possible to find value in illness that either lingers on as chronic or ends in death? The answer seems to be in focusing less on recovery and more on renewal.

Arthur Frank, PhD

After the diagnosis of a severe or life-threatening illness, people face the daunting task of dealing with daily stress and uncertainty, reorganizing their life and relationships, and moving on to find happiness in a changed and sometimes more physically limited life. Over time, they must work to maintain or rebuild their self-confidence and self-worth, their relationships, and find purpose, peace, and happiness in day-to-day life.

How do people who are diagnosed with a serious illness get through each day, cope with stress, and start their recovery? What helps them to regain a life that has value to them? Several themes emerge from conversations with patients and the memoirs of people who have written about illness.

THE ROLE OF A SPIRITUAL LIFE
Although few people report that they "find God" during the stress of their illness, those who believe in God often find tremendous support in that relationship and in their relationship with the clergy and the community of people with whom they worship. Religious beliefs about the meaning of life, suffering, and the afterlife offer consolation to those who are ill. In

the conversation of prayer and their relationship with God, isolation and vulnerability lessen. Tom Moran developed AIDS when there were few effective treatments available. He wrote about prayer as follows:

> But the private part of it, the prayer, matters most of all. And as far as prayer goes, you know, the more you pray, the stronger your prayers, the more fixed your heart and your mind are. And I am finding that to be very refreshing. And very good. Especially my moments when I despair. And I lose faith. And I lose courage. And I lose hope. What helps the most then is to pray, like they often do chants in other cultures. . . . There is great strength in that, and it really does help me to find centeredness, and the light of God and the strength of God in my life.
>
> *Tom Moran*, People with AIDS

People who do not have strong religious beliefs still find comfort and a way to deal with uncertainty, anxiety, and sadness in a spiritual life. For many, spending time out of doors in the quiet and beauty of nature provides peace and solace. Fitzhugh Mullan wrote:

> As my illness progressed I wondered if my attitude about God and religion would change. Would I, faced with the prospect of death, find a piety or belief that had not been apparent in health? That did not happen. I grappled with my fate without benefit or burden of religious belief. It is hard to know whether it is good or bad, but it was natural for me. I think that while my experience with illness has made me more spiritual – teaching me, as it has, greater respect for the richness as well as the frailty of life – it has not made me more religious. To me it was the struggle of a human spirit and a human body.

Quiet walks, alone or with others, help to calm anxiety and provide time to refocus and rethink priorities, goals, and values. Regular walks were an important part of Arthur Frank's recovery:

> I still needed time myself. . . . I chose the time for these walks so that I would come over the crest of the hill just as the afternoon sun shone directly on the water. . . . I wanted to store up these elements against the possibility that I might be deprived of them. In that sunlight in the river I began to heal.

Ted Kooser, the 13th US Poet Laureate, found that he was anxious, depressed, and unable to write during his treatment for squamous-cell cancer of the tongue. In this excerpt from an essay he wrote about his illness, he talks about the importance of his daily walk during his cancer treatment:

. . . On Monday we met my surgeon, a pleasant but serious young man who asked if I had any public speaking in my work. He'd have to remove part of my tongue, and I might have a speech problem. "No speaking that I can't live without", I said. Kathleen interrupted and said, "But he is a poet, he gives poetry readings." By the time we saw him again, he had been to the public library, checked out my books, and read them.

Surgery followed. My doctor had expected the tumor to be early in its development, confined to the site, but he did a neck dissection to be sure it hadn't spread. It had, to the upper lymph nodes under my jaw. He told me this bad news in my room at the hospital, recommended a full course of radiation, and then, when his clutch of young residents had moved into the hall, stayed behind for a moment. "I don't know what kind of spiritual life you have, Mr. Kooser", he said, "but you are about to enter one of the greatest life-affirming experiences."

Five days a week for 6 weeks I reported to a Lincoln hospital for radiation. My mouth erupted in sores that persisted for weeks after I completed the treatments. I could only eat milkshakes and Ensure. Each day when I came home, I stopped at the head of our lane and picked up a pebble from the road. I lined these up along the kitchen windowsill to count off the treatments. It took a lifetime, it seemed, to get to thirty. I dreaded waking up in the morning.

From the first of June 'til early winter, I was exhausted, anxious, depressed, and unable to write. I began taking a 2-mile walk each morning. I had been told to stay out of the sun for a year because of skin sensitivity, so I exercised before dawn, hiking the isolated country roads near where I live, sometimes with my wife, but often alone.

Then, as autumn began to fade and winter came on, I began to heal. One morning in early November, following my walk, I surprised myself by writing a poem. Soon, I was writing every morning. . . . I wrote 130 poems that winter. . . . God had taken my Donkey and helped me find it again. You never know.

CREATING A NEW LIFE

Some people fully recover from serious illness and go back to the life they used to live, usually with different perspectives. However, many cannot go back. Eventually they have to deal with the reality that they will have to create a new purpose in life, a reason to get up in the morning, a schedule, a new routine. The decision to give up the hope of being able to go back to the life you used to live – your work, your family roles, your hobbies – is a wrenching one. And finding the motivation to move on may be even more difficult. Reynolds Price counseled people facing serious illness to find meaningful ways to occupy their time, and to return to any kind of work that gives structure to the day, distraction from worries, relationships in the outside world, and a sense of identity – this is who I am, this is what I do. Above all, he advised them not to sit passively waiting for the old life to return or to insist that nothing short of the old life would be adequate.

> Being ill is just another way of living.
>
> ARTHUR FRANK, PHD

The stunned hours of blank wall gazing that eagerly await you . . . find any legal way to avoid my first mistake which was to sit still in cooperation. . . . Play cut-throat card games, leave the house when you can, go sit in the park near children at play, read to children in a cancer ward, go donate whatever strength you've got to feeding the hungry or tending the millions worse off than you. I wish to God I had – any legal acts to break the inward gaze at my withering self.

. . . Generous people – true practical saints, some of them boring as root canals – are waiting to give you everything on earth but your main want, which is simply the person you used to be. . . . Grieve for a decent limited time over whatever parts of your old self you know you'll miss. . . . The kindest thing that anyone could have done for me, once I'd finished 5 weeks of radiation, would have been to look me squarely in the eye and say this clearly, "Reynolds Price is dead. Who will you be now? Who can you be and how can you get there, double time?" . . . Come back to life, whoever you'll be. Only you can do it.

. . . [The] basic point for cancer patients – or, for that matter, for everyone – is a simple and good one. Live the life you have left and don't wallow in memories and speculations about what life might have been or ought to be.

Because work is such an important part of our identity and occupies so much of the day, return to work is a major part of recovery for people who are well enough to try – even if they return to a job that was previously boring or stressful. At the very minimum, it provides a distraction. It forces you to get up in the morning and gives structure and routine to the day. And for many it is much more than that – it restores a sense of purpose. Being out of work and living on disability income, even if this is initially welcome, can be demoralizing. Fitzhugh Mullan found that his return to the routine of work, although exhausting and anxiety producing, was an important way to restart and refocus his life:

> The first day [at work] was horrible. I had no clothes that fit me. It was one thing to loll around the house in baggy trousers and shirts hopelessly stooped at the shoulders, but it was another to enter the competitive world of officer workers looking like a refugee. I had intended to work until noon, but by mid morning I was feeling ill and my head was swimming. I escaped to the cubicle assigned to me to rest my head on the desk until I had significant energy to plot my trip home. . . . Things did improve. . . . My new-found usefulness proved to be an essential factor in helping me re-establish my identity as a worker, breadwinner, and doctor. Week by week I became more enthusiastic about the job. . . . The more involved I became with work, the healthier I felt in my mind.

It can take years to return to work or to re-establish a daily routine that gives focus and meaning to the day. People in physically demanding jobs are often never able to return to work. Limited resources, transportation, and education make it much more challenging to find work after disability. However, they can often find new roles, volunteering in the community or mentoring or becoming involved with a child or young adult who needs advice and guidance.

REDEVELOPING RELATIONSHIPS WITH FAMILY AND FRIENDS

Relationships with family and friends can change dramatically during illness. However, there is no time in life when close relationships are more important, as they provide the physical and emotional support that sustains people through critical illness. When you are ill you need a cadre of friends who will rally to your side – friends who will sit with you, listen to you, console you, offer to help, make you laugh, and distract you. The relationships with these people are often permanently strengthened.

However, many people don't really understand the personal impact of illness and don't always offer appropriate help and support. Disappointment with those friends, family members and co-workers can lead to temporary or permanent estrangement and contributes to a sense of isolation. Arthur Frank wrote about his friendships as follows:

> I have two friends who have abandoned me since I had AIDS. AIDS is like any other disease, and some people just don't deal with sickness very well. I don't think these two friends have abandoned me because I have AIDS. I think they just can't cope with illness of any sort.
>
> PAUL FOWLER,
> *PEOPLE WITH AIDS*

> Some came through; others disappeared. We now find it hard to resume relationships with those who could not acknowledge the illness that was happening, not just to me but to us. Those relationships were a loss.
>
> *Arthur Frank, PhD*

In his book, Reynolds Price wrote extensively about the unselfish and unfailing support of his friends. Arthur Frank and Fitzhugh Mullan wrote that their relationships with their wives sustained them through the most difficult parts of their illnesses:

> I was glad for having done the things I had done, for having a daughter who would have some memories of her father, a wife to whom I had given some pleasure, and parents to whom I had given some pride. I had practiced medicine for six years and had, I hoped, given benefit to a number of patients. . . . That was my tally sheet, and in stoic moments I was happy with it.
>
> *Fitzhugh Mullen, MD*

Many patients say that their relationship with children – a grandchild or their own children – was a tremendous source of hope, affection, and distraction during illness. Young children are nonjudgmental (especially about appearances), physically affectionate (at a time when the patient might not be feeling attractive or finding other sources of affection), and help them to find joy in the world.

DETERMINATION AND HOPE

Adjustment to the new realities of life with illness takes time, but time moves excruciatingly slowly after the diagnosis of serious illness and during treatment. Waiting for test results, recovering from surgery, dealing with the side-effects of treatment that leave people feeling so fatigued or nauseated that they can't enjoy a family meal, or sitting at home for hours without being able to accomplish anything – all of these things make people feel that life is happening in slow motion. Getting through each day is one of the most difficult challenges. In the end, it is the ability to just go on – to put one foot in front of the other and live each day – that starts recovery.

> The struggle for me in my medical gulag was never a question of bravery or heroism. Doggedness is what it took to survive – drab, stolid, life-sustaining doggedness.
>
> *Fitzhugh Mullan, MD*

> I take my life day to day. Just day to day.
>
> *Paul Fowler,* People with AIDS

The determination to move on is supported by hope – hope that there may eventually be a treatment or a cure, hope that an acceptable life can be rebuilt, hope that, if there is no effective treatment, family, friends, and physicians will do everything possible to maximize one's quality of life and dignity. Hope is the force that keeps people moving forward during illness. Without it, it is hard to motivate patients to comply with treatment and to put up with the challenges that modern medical care imposes:

Last fall I planted 200 various and sundry bulbs in my garden. Most of which are coming up this year. You take your chances. And you hope. You do hope. And, in fact, I've planted my bulbs for later this summer. You do the best you can and you go on. I think that's what human beings do. Some of us unfortunately have been given a few extra factors to struggle with. AIDS is an extra factor to struggle with.

Paul Fowler, People with AIDS

Aftermath: Life after Illness

. . . the ultimate value of illness is that it teaches us the value of being
alive.

Arthur Frank, PhD

NEW PERSPECTIVES

Illness – and the associated fatigue, physical disability and time needed
away from home and work for testing and treatment – slows the pace of life
and forces you out of the routine of the life you used to live. While the loss
of that routine can be disturbing, it also offers opportunities for unhurried
observation and time to examine the essential elements of life that bring
happiness and meaning. Although few people say that their illness has made
them a different person, it can change one's outlook on life. Many people
become more patient, reflective, and appreciative of small things. They re-
examine personal relationships and their values and professional goals.

Arthur Frank and Fitzhugh Mullan describe how illness changed their
goals and their values:

> Critical illness offers the opportunity to be taken to the threshold of life,
> from which you can see where your life could end. From that vantage point
> you are both forced and allowed to think in new ways about the value of
> life. Alive but detached from everyday living, you can finally stop to consider

why you have lived as you have and what future you would like, if any future is possible. Illness takes away parts of your life, but in doing so gives you the opportunity to choose the life you will lead as opposed to living out the one you have simply accumulated over the years.

. . . My life had not stopped, but a great deal of it had been put on hold. Now I could begin to make plans again, to think of travel, to commit myself to projects at work. The process of re-entry was not smooth. I now knew that the way that I and others lived was a choice, and often not the best one. My consciousness remained suspended between the insulated world of illness and the "healthy" mainstream. This suspension expressed itself in lack of tolerance for tension and disagreements. I continued to value much of the life of an ill person, even though I was no longer officially diseased.

. . . The only real difference between people is not health or illness, but the way each holds on to a sense of value in life. When I feel I have no time to walk out and watch the sunlight on the river, my recovery has gone too far. A little fear is all right. . . . When the ordinary is frustrating, I have to remember those times when the ordinary was forbidden to me. When I was ill, all that I wanted was to get back to the ordinary flux of activity. Now that I am back in the ordinary, I have to retain a sense of wonder at being there.

. . . Recovery has different meanings. After my heart attack it meant putting the whole experience behind me. I wanted to return to a place in the healthy mainstream as if nothing had happened. Cancer does not allow that version of recovery. I am reminded, every time I see a doctor or fill out an insurance form, that there is no "cure" for cancer, only remission. But more important than the physiology of disease is the impact of the experience. After cancer, I had no desire to go back to where I was before. The opportunity for change had been purchased at too great a cost to let it slip away. I had seen too much suffering from a perspective that is often invisible to the young and the healthy. I could not take up the same game on the old terms. I wanted less to recover what I had been than to discover what else I might be.

Arthur Frank, PhD

Throughout this period I was pursued by a nagging expectation. I anticipated being a different person after what I had been through. I had come so close to death that I imagined my perspective on life would be different. I fantasized that certain personal pettinesses of mine would disappear and that I would be wiser and more temperate than I had been before. . . . Much to my dismay, things were not different. As far as I could tell, I responded and behaved much as I always had. I was neither missionary nor saint. The egocentricities that had been mine a year earlier had survived the ordeal intact. My personality was alive and passably well, but it was definitely not "born again."

. . . In no way do I mean to recommend or endorse serious sickness, but living through it has, I think, left me with a fuller sense of life. This sense includes the inevitability of death attended by some quantity of pain and despair as well as the richness of life in the years that are ours. . . . Sometimes in the bustle of rekindled life, amidst the demands, the distractions, and the fatigue, I forget how good those things really are and how easily they might not have been. That is a simple message and a happy one – and one that I am delighted to be able to share.

Fitzhugh Mullan, MD

Dr. Harvey Mandell's diagnosis and treatment for melanoma refocused his ideas about what is important in life:

Living a met free existence helps me to put a lot of thing into perspective. Trivia that might ordinarily consume you are easily set aside or even ignored. What people think of you becomes of little importance as long as you are convinced that you are doing the right thing and as long as the few people in the world whose opinions are important to you agree. You don't become saintly or even necessarily a great guy, but you do learn to tune out a lot of unimportant matters.

RESIDUAL EFFECTS

Visit after visit, when I walk through the door to see Mr. Percy, the engineer with dermatomyositis, I am relieved to see his level of recovery. He is much better now – off oxygen, except when he exercises, and off corticosteroid medications. He is back to his old job, golfs with a cart occasionally, and although he no longer travels to dog shows, he is able to keep his dogs at his home again.

I have asked him a number of times if he would talk to a group of medical students about the personal impact of his illness, and his response was always the same – "In a few more months, I just need a little more time" he says, looking away. At his routine office visits, when I inquire how he is doing, he usually replies – "Not great", or "Terrible" or, at best, "I'm still here." Recently, I asked him how he felt about his life now that the disease was controlled. He looked down, shook his head and said, simply, that he thought his life would never be the same and that he would never feel that he was safe again. His social life is very limited, he doesn't sleep well, and he finds it difficult to motivate himself to exercise and manage his weight, even though he knows that doing both is critical for controlling his diabetes.

While recovery can lead to a new appreciation of life, serious illness exposes people, sometimes for the first time, to a more pessimistic view of life, their relationships, and their future, and can have permanent psychological effects. Arthur Kleinman wrote:

> The moral lesson illness teaches us is that there are undesired and undeserved pains that must be lived through, that beneath the façade of blind optimism regarding the natural order of things, there is a deeper apprehension of a dark hurtful stream of negative events and troubles. Change, caprice, and chaos experienced in the body challenge what order we are led to believe – need to believe – exists.

I now realize that I will never have a single conclusion about my cancer. . . . It is with me for the rest of my life. For better and for worse, I will live with it and quietly work and rework my personal history in an effort to accommodate it as much as possible.

FITZHUGH MULLAN, MD

When a patient's disease comes under control or goes into remission, they return to their previous life – as imperfect as it may have been – but they are often not the same person. The emotional trauma of the illness, the failure of their body to function as they expected it would, the damage to their self-image and relationships, and the flaws that they had to deal with in the medical system may leave them with grimmer expectations and a more cynical outlook on life. Their personal and professional life may be permanently damaged.

Physicians are sometimes surprised or annoyed by patients who continue to be preoccupied with their bodily symptoms well after recovery. While we are delighted and relieved when the disease is under control, we may find that the patient's complaints increase. They don't share our optimism and relief that it is "all over." Anxiety and depression can prevent them from re-establishing relationships and a daily routine, returning to work, or planning for the future – even when the illness is in remission or is cured. Disability can lead to deconditioning, which worsens anxiety and sleeplessness. Often neither the patient nor the physician recognizes that complaints of fatigue, sleeplessness, loss of appetite, inability to exercise and lack of motivation may be signs of anxiety and depression. And, even when recognized, they are frequently difficult to treat.

Other patients may be much more successful at keeping their anxiety, sorrow, worry, and depression to themselves. An oncologist told me the story of a young woman who showed remarkable determination and an upbeat attitude during surgery, radiation, and chemotherapy for sarcoma. At a routine visit after the successful completion of her treatment, she smiled and talked calmly about the future follow-up plans. It was not until her doctor got up to leave that she said, "Can I ask you a question?" As her face fell she started to cry and said "I think about the cancer all the time. I worry about it every day. At work, they asked me to talk to a co-worker who has cancer because they see me as a survivor. But I don't want to talk to her. I don't feel like a survivor and I can't stand to talk about cancer."

The oncologist was completely taken aback by her comments. The young woman had never given any clues about her anxiety. Often doctors find that it is difficult to judge how a patient is dealing with illness by their outward appearance. The most cheerful or apparently calm person can be suffering. You don't know unless you ask.

Arthur Frank has written extensively about the psychological aftermath of his illness. In the excerpts that follow he describes how every test or visit to the doctor reminds him that he will always be a patient, how the fear brought on by the vulnerability lingers for years into recovery,

> Though the scars are the most graphic reminder of the past, there are dozens of other ligatures that keep me tethered to the cancer experience. Behind every cough, cold, ache, and pain there lurks the ghost of seminoma.
>
> FITZHUGH MULLAN, MD

and that the illness of others reminds him of his own vulnerability:

> I have learned that the changes that begin during illness do not end when treatment stops. Life after critical illness does not go back to where it was before. . . . And those ill persons who recover must recover not only from the disease but also from being a patient.
>
> . . . I become less and less a person with cancer, but the continuing schedule of examination, X-rays and blood tests reminds me that I am at greater risk than others. This risk diminishes over time but never disappears. . . . No matter how well I had insulated myself with the concerns of work and home, my monthly pilgrimage to the oncology clinic would remind me of the tenuous nature of my "cure."
>
> . . . I am trying, in this third year after cancer, to be a little less afraid.
>
> . . . I still feel threatened by disease and the suffering of others. . . . I fear not only suffering but slowing down.

Dr. Eric Cassel wrote about this vulnerable period:

> In many chronic or serious diseases, persons who "recover" or who seem successfully treated do not return to normal function. They may never again be employed, recover sexual function, pursue career goals, re-establish family relationships, or re-enter the social world despite a physical cure. Such patients may not have recovered from the nonphysical changes occurring with physical illness. It should come as no surprise, then, that chronic suffering frequently follows in the wake of disease.

In the excerpts that follow, Fitzhugh Mullan describes the change in his approach to life and people after his illness:

> But, over time, I have done a lot of grieving for the future on the chance that I may not be there. That is a strange way to spend time and emotion . . .
>
> As I became more active professionally and socially, I would meet people who I had known previously. It was impossible to know how to respond to the simple query "How have you been?". The answer "fine" was not true. "Pretty good except for a touch of cancer" was not good either. While I was not averse to sharing my experience, I had neither the time nor the energy to share them with casual acquaintances.

Jane Kenyon, a poet who had an extended remission from breast cancer, wrote about the joy of returning to the day-to-day activities that she had taken for granted, after successful treatment. And in the midst of the following poem about the triumph of survival, she also captures the lingering sense of vulnerability:

Otherwise

I got out of bed
on two strong legs.
It might have been
otherwise. I ate
cereal, sweet
milk, ripe flawless
peach. It might
have been otherwise.
I took the dog uphill
to the birch wood.
All morning I did
the work I love.

At noon I lay down
with my mate. It might
have been otherwise.
We ate dinner together
at a table with silver
candlesticks. It might
have been otherwise.

I slept in a bed
in a room with paintings
on the walls, and
planned another day
just like this day.
But one day, I know,
it will be otherwise.

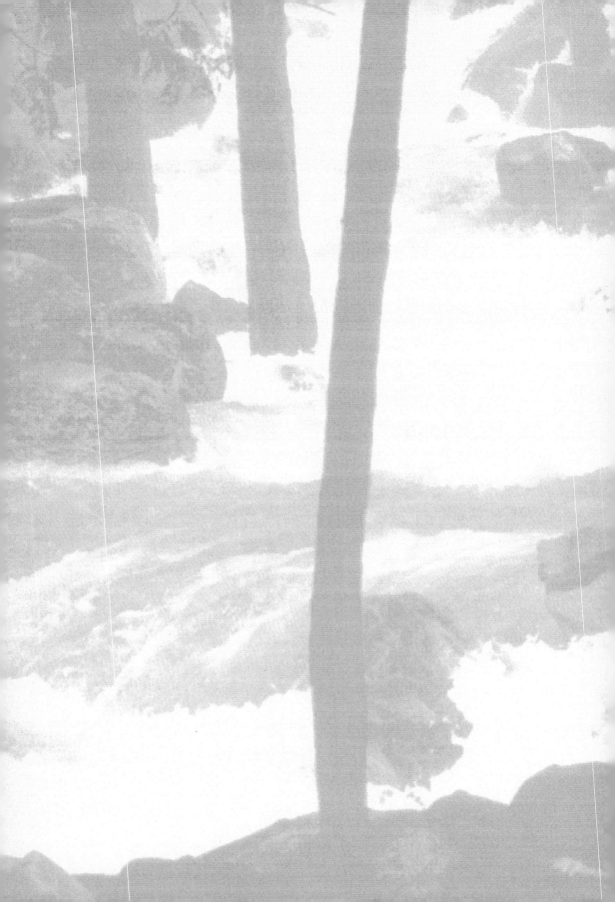

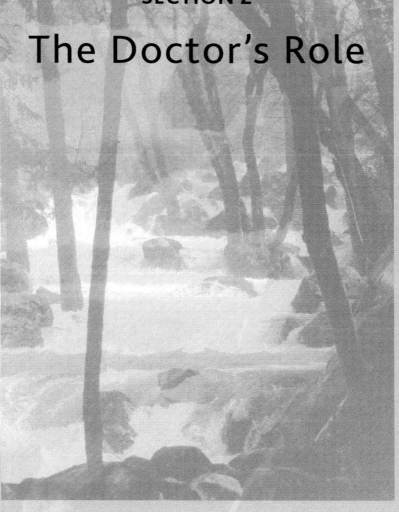

SECTION 2

The Doctor's Role

There, I think, is the oldest and most effective act of doctors, the touching. Some people don't like being handled by others, but not, or almost never, sick people. They need being touched, and part of the dismay in being very sick is the lack of close human contact. Ordinary people, even close friends, even family members, tend to stay away from the very sick, touching them as infrequently as possible for fear of interfering, or catching the illness, or just fear of bad luck. The doctor's oldest skill in trade was to place his hands on the patient.

Lewis Thomas, MD

This patient . . . edified me about the experience of illness and the doctor's attention to disease – a key distinction.

Arthur Kleinman, MD

Empathy and Compassion

Empathy, however, underlies the qualities of the humanistic physician and should frame the skills of all professionals who care for patients.

Howard Spiro, MD

Empathy – the ability to identify with and understand another person's experience – facilitates most human relationships. Studies show that one of the predictors of empathetic behavior in physicians is whether they have been personally affected by illness – either themselves or through a close relationship. That experience opens their eyes to the personal impact of illness and the difficulties inherent in dealing with the medical bureaucracy.

Identifying with a person, seeing them as someone like you, facilitates empathy. However, there are significant institutional barriers to empathy, and the setting in which we provide care is one of them. In small communities, where doctors live and interact with their patients day to day, they are more likely to see their patient as a whole person – in all their roles – and to know their family. But the practice of medicine is increasingly complex and, for efficiency, care is delivered in centralized facilities. In these less personal settings, we rarely get a sense of the patient as a person, and their psychosocial problems are often well hidden.

When a person is hospitalized, they become a patient – transformed by the hospital environment and the nondescript gown that they wear into someone who is different from the rest of us and different from the person they have been. There they are deprived of the simple things that comfort them and remind them of who they are – a warm private shower or the clothes that give them a sense of their identity, as well as dignity. Most of us spend a good deal of time in the morning showering and dressing in a way that conveys the image we want to project to the world. Imagine if you arrived at work or a social situation unbathed, with your hair uncombed, in a nondescript tunic (no pants of course), with slippers on. This is the attire in which hospitalized patients will conduct some of the most important interactions of their life – communicating with healthcare providers to optimize their health. The attire alone reinforces the image of the patient as a passive participant rather than an independent, unique, and competent person.

The physical environment of the hospital does not promote empathy or personal conversations. The colors are usually drab or, at best, institutional, the environment is noisy, the staff are rushed, and it is usually difficult for physicians and patients to find private space to sit and talk. Most rooms have two people and, even in private rooms, there is an endless stream of medical personnel walking through the room unannounced.

Care for the hospitalized patient is frequently provided by a new physician – the hospitalist – with whom the patient usually has no pre-existing relationship. As the hospitalist is pressured to treat and discharge patients quickly, time spent getting to know the patient as a person may seem like an unnecessary luxury.

I suppose that over the past 30 years I have counseled over 500 students wishing to discuss a career in medicine. No one has ever asked, "Do I have enough empathy to be a health professional?" Hundreds have asked, "Do I have high enough grades in organic chemistry or high enough MCATs to get into medical school?"

HAROLD MOROWITZ

Time is a barrier to empathy. During training and in practice, great value is placed on endurance and the ability to work long hours. A recent study found that the natural empathy of first year medical students decreases during their training, weakened by the culture, environment, and time demands of undergraduate medical education. Fatigue does not promote empathy. Doctors who are rushed or overworked just try to get the basics done. Empathy erodes slowly, and most of us never recognize the change in our interactions with patients.

The complexity of modern medical care has diffused the personal relationships between physicians and patients that led to empathy.

Fifty years ago, diagnoses were made by careful examination and repeated bedside interactions with and observations of patients by a small group of providers. Now, technology is more likely to provide the diagnoses, not time spent with patients. The doctors are clustered around computers in team rooms, ordering tests and reviewing results. Time spent interacting with patients is limited.

The team approach to care, which involves trainees, consultants, and proceduralists, increases the expertise and oversight given to increasingly complex medical treatment, but can also interfere with empathy. It is often unclear who is responsible for educating and counseling the patient. Is it the resident, who has the least understanding of the personal impact of illness? Is it the supervising physician, who spends the least time with the patient? Or is it the consulting physician who makes the diagnosis and treatment recommendations? Is it the nurse's job? But, the most skilled nurses – those with the best understanding of illness – are usually dispensing medication and providing critical bedside care. With shared responsibility, the rush of hospitalization and testing, and the complexity of the work to be done, little time is spent in the room with the patient establishing a relationship and discussing the implications of the diagnosis. Unless some psychosocial issue gets in the way of discharge, patients are usually sent home with little or no time spent educating them about the illness, its potential impact on their life, and their role in controlling it.

Many of us train in inner-city or state hospitals that provide care for the poor and uninsured. Tired and rushed, residents and students often find themselves frustrated with patients who don't appear to be motivated to improve their health, or grateful for the care that they receive. There is a wide separation between the lives of these busy, upwardly mobile physicians in training and their ill patients who are vulnerable, discouraged, powerless, frequently passive, and sometimes hostile.

Dan Gilbert, a psychologist, researcher, and author, argues that much of human happiness comes from thinking about and planning for the future – anticipating new relationships, career opportunities, experiences, and possessions that will make life "complete." Feeling that you have some control over the direction of your life is critical to that anticipation. Physicians in training are at the peak of planning and anticipation of their future life and, in general, are "take control" people with the resources – education, anticipated income, and personal support – to try to effect that change. However, many of the people we treat, especially those who have not had the same opportunities and resources, live a life over which they have little control and, at some point, they may stop trying. Serious illness adds to that vulnerability, lack of control, and inability to plan for the future. It is not surprising that some patients face illness with the same passivity with which they live their life. They may no longer believe that they can impact the direction of their life or envision a better life.

So physicians who are actively building a life may have trouble identifying with or understanding the life of their patients – a life that is often in disarray and without clear direction or motivation. However, without that identification, it is difficult to be empathetic. In *Medicine as a Human Experience*, Drs. Reiser and Rosen remind us of the common humanity we share with these patients:

> Conversation helps to develop empathy, for it is here that we learn of shared experience and feelings.
>
> HOWARD SPIRO, MD,
> *EMPATHY AND THE PRACTICE OF MEDICINE*

Even the most isolated, down-and-out skid-row derelict has a life. He must have a place somewhere where he hangs out, and usually there are people he hangs out with; moreover, there are assuredly things that matter to him – maybe just a soiled snapshot or a tattered address book. Above all, everyone has memories and a past. Everyone had a mother and a father – once. Everyone also has a future – hopes, aspirations, dreams – these as well as illnesses and fears. Even our most anonymous patients have a life. Students should never forget that hospitals are very artificial environments. Hospitalized patients are stripped of their clothing, their wallets, and their jewelry. Favorite pipes and pictures are gone. We tell them to lie down flat. We isolate them from so much that makes each of them a person. Why we do this is both curious and complex. In some ways it seems necessary. Sometimes one wonders, though. . . . Whatever the reason for our rituals, remember that the supine figure that you see on the gurney under the sheet has a life, as surely as you or I. It is always worth enquiring into, for it is virtually impossible to treat someone despicably whom one understands, and sometimes our understanding itself can help immeasurably.

As careers in medicine progress, personal, financial, regulatory, and professional forces often pull physicians away from the original motivation and values that led them to choose medicine as their profession. Many doctors feel that their personal relationship with their patients – those conversations about family and personal aspirations, shared laughter, and grief over losses – sustains their interest in the practice of medicine and prevents burnout. These conversations take surprisingly little time and, over years of practice, come together to form a composite that gives a fuller picture of the patient as a person like you. The insights that come from relationships with patients give meaning and interest to practice, day in and day out, in an era of increasing bureaucracy and technology.

> Whenever I hear a certain reluctance on the part of my house staff to discuss or see a patient, or when I hear the words "placement problem", I worry that we are dealing with a story that has not found its epiphany. The challenge is to enter that room despite the magnetic draw of beepers pulling us away and the seemingly more urgent needs of other patients. The challenge is to engage the patient and the family and find the epiphany, even if the epiphany is simply that there is nothing more that can be done medically. The epiphany might simply be a coming to terms with the illness by all concerned – patient, family, and doctors.
>
> *Abraham Verghese*, The Physician as Storyteller

In the literature of medicine, there is a steadily growing interest in the narrative aspects of medical practice and physicians' writings about their work. Underlying this interest is the assumption that careful attention to the language and stories of medicine can enrich the doctor–patient relationship, improve patient care, and enhance doctors' sense of satisfaction with their work.

> When internists were asked to write about a work experience that was important, fulfilling, or reaffirmed their commitment to medicine, one major theme that emerged was making a connection with their patient. A growing body of research shows that the patient–physician relationship is the most consistently reported and powerful determinant of physician satisfaction.
>
> *Carol R. Horowitz* et al.

This section on empathy ends with excerpts from the essays of Lewis Thomas, MD (1913–1993), a researcher and writer who published a series of essays in the *New England Journal of Medicine*, and William Carlos Williams, MD (1883–1963), a family practitioner in a poor area of New Jersey at the turn of the century, and a renowned poet. Both men describe how empathy and relationships with patients were at the core of a satisfying career in medicine.

Lewis Thomas, *The Youngest Science*, Chapter 20: Illness

One of the hard things to learn in medicine, even harder to teach, is what it feels like to be a patient. In the old days, when serious illness was a more commonplace experience, shared round by everyone, the doctor had usually been through at least a few personal episodes on his own and had a pretty good idea of what it was like for his patient. A good many of the specialists in pulmonary disease who were brought up in the early years of this century had first acquired their interest in the field from having had tuberculosis themselves. Some of the leading figures in rehabilitation medicine had been crippled by poliomyelitis. And all physicians of those generations knew about pneumonia and typhoid at first hand, or at least once removed, in themselves or their immediate families.

It is very different today. The killing or near-killing illnesses are largely reserved for one's advanced years. No one goes through the six or eight perilous weeks of typhoid anymore, coming within sight of dying every day, getting through at the end with a stronger character perhaps, certainly with a different way of looking at life. The high technologies which are turned on to cope with serious disease – the electronic monitoring in intensive care, the chemotherapy drugs for cancer, the tour de force accomplishments of contemporary surgery, and the mobilization of increasingly complex procedures for diagnosis in medicine – are matters to be mastered only from lecture notes and books, and then by actual practice on patients, but very few doctors have more than an inkling of what it is actually like to go through such experiences. Even the childhood contagions are mostly gone, thanks to vaccines for measles, whooping cough, chickenpox, and the like, thanks especially to the easy control of streptococcal infections. Today's young doctors do not know what it is like to have an earache, much less what it is like to have an eardrum punctured.

The nearest thing to a personal education in illness is the grippe. It is almost all we have left in the way of on-the-job training, and I hope that somehow it can be spared as we proceed to eliminate so many other human diseases. Indeed, I would favor hanging on to the grippe, and its cousin the common cold, for as long as possible. A case could be made, I think, for viewing the various viruses involved in these minor but impressive illnesses as a set of endangered species, essentially good for the human environment, something like snail darters.

Most people afflicted with the grippe complain about it, and that is one of its virtues. It is good for people to have, from time to time, something to complain about, a genuine demon. It is a good thing to be laid up once in a while, compelled by nature to stop doing whatever else and to take to bed. It is an especially good thing to have a fever and the malaise that goes with fever, when you know that it will be gone in three or four days but meanwhile entitles you to all the privileges of the sick: bed rest, ice water on the bed table, aspirin, maybe an ice bag on the head or behind the neck, and the attentions of one's solicitous family. Sympathy: how many other opportunities turn up in a lifetime to engage the sympathy and concern of others for something that is not your fault and will surely be gone in a few days? Preserve the grippe, I say, and find some way to insert it into the practical curriculum of all medical students. Twice a year, say, the lecture hall in molecular biochemistry should be exposed to a silent aerosol of adenovirus, so that the whole class comes down at once. Schedules being what they are in medical schools, this will assure that a good many students will be obliged to stay on their feet, working through the next days and nights with their muscle pains and fever, and learning what it is like *not* to be cared for. Good for them, and in a minor way good for their future as doctors.

In another essay, Lewis Thomas counsels medical students about the future of medicine and relationship with patients (Chapter 6: Leech Leech, Et Cetera):

Today, the doctor can perform a great many of his most essential tasks from his office in another building without ever seeing the patient. There are even computer programs for taking a history: a clerk can ask the questions and check the boxes on a printed form, and the computer will instantly provide a printout of the diagnostic possibilities to be considered and the laboratory procedures to be undertaken. Instead of spending forty-five minutes listening to the chest and palpating the abdomen, the doctor can sign a slip which sends the patient off to the X-ray department for a CT scan, with the expectation of seeing within the hour, in exquisite detail, all the body's internal organs which he formerly had to make guesses about with his fingers and ears. The biochemistry laboratory eliminates the need for pondering and waiting for the appearances of new signs and symptoms. Computerized devices reveal electronic intimacies of the flawed heart or malfunctioning of the brain with a precision far beyond the touch or reach, or even the imagining, of the physician at the bedside a few generations back.

The doctor can set himself, if he likes, at a distance remote from the patient and the family, never touching anyone beyond a perfunctory hand-shake as the first and only contact. Medicine is no longer a laying on of hands, it is more like the reading of signals from machines.

The mechanism of scientific medicine is here to stay. The new medicine works. It is a vastly more complicated profession, with more things to be done at short notice on which issues of life or death depend. The physician has the same obligations that he carried, overworked and often despair-ingly, fifty years ago, but now with a number of technological maneuvers to be undertaken quickly and with precision. It looks to the patient like a different experience from what his parents told him about, with something important left out. The doctor seems less like a close friend and confidant, less interested in him as a person, wholly concerned with treating the disease. And there is no changing this, no going back; nor, when you think about it, is there really any reason for wanting to go back. If I develop the signs and symptoms of malignant hypertension, or cancer of the colon, or subacute bacterial endocarditis, I want as much comfort and friendship as I can find at hand, but mostly I want to be treated quickly and effectively so as to survive, if that is possible. If I am in bed in a modern hospital, worry-ing about the cost of that bed as well, I want to get out as fast as possible, whole if possible.

In my father's time, talking with the patient was the biggest part of medicine, for that was almost all there was to do. The doctor–patient relationship was, for better or worse, a long conversation in which the patient was the epicenter of concern and knew it. When I was an intern and scientific technology was in its earliest stage, the talk was still there, but hurried, often on the run.

Today, with the advance of medicine's various and complicated new technologies, the ward rounds are not at the foot of the bed, the drawing of blood samples for automated assessment of every known (or suggested) biochemical abnormality, the rolling of wheelchairs and litters down the corridors to the X-ray department, there is less time for talking. The longest and most personal conversations held with hospitalized patients when they come in the hospital are discussions of finances and insurance, engaged in by personnel trained in accountancy, whose scientific instruments are the computers. The hospitalized patient feels, for a time, like a working part of an immense, automated apparatus. He is admitted and discharged by batteries of computers, sometimes without even learning the doctors' names. The difference may be strange and vaguely dismaying for patients. But there is another difference, worth emphasis. Many of the patients go home speedily and in good health, cured of their disease. In my father's day, this happened much less often, and when it did, it was a matter of good luck or a strong constitution. When it happens today, it is more frequently due to technology.

There are costs to be faced. Not just money, the real and heavy dollar costs. The close up, reassuring, warm touch of the physician, the comfort and concern, the long, leisurely discussion in which everything including the dog can be worked into the conversation, are disappearing from the practice of medicine, and this may turn out to be too great a loss for the doctor as well as for the patient. This uniquely subtle, personal relationship has roots that go back into the beginnings of medicine's history, and needs preserving. To do it right has never been easy; it takes the best doctors, the best of friends. Once lost, even for as short a time as one generation, it may be too difficult a task to bring it back again.

If I were a medical student or an intern, just getting ready to begin, I would be more worried about this aspect of my future than anything else. I would be apprehensive that my real job, caring for sick people, might soon be taken away, leaving me with the quite different occupation of looking after machines. I would be trying to figure out ways to keep this from happening.

William Carlos Williams, MD, The Practice (from *The Autobiography*)

It's the humdrum, day-in, day-out, everyday work that is the real satisfaction of the practice of medicine; the million and a half visits that a man has seen on his daily visits over a forty-year period of weekdays and Sundays that make up his life. I have never had a money practice; it would have been impossible for me. But the actual calling on people at all times and under all conditions, the coming to grips with the intimate condition of their lives, when they were being born, when they were dying, watching them die, watching them get well when they were ill, has always absorbed me.

I lost myself in the very properties of their minds: for the moment at least I actually became them, whoever they should be, so that when I detached myself from them at the end of a half-hour of intense concentration over some illness which was affecting them, it was as though I was awakening from sleep. For the moment I myself did not exist, nothing of myself affected me. As a consequence I came back to myself, as from any other sleep, rested.

Time after time I have gone out into my office in the evening feeling as if I couldn't keep my eyes open a moment longer. I would start out on my morning calls after only a few hours sleep, sit in front of some house waiting to get the courage to climb the steps and push the front-door bell. But once I saw the patient all that would disappear. In a flash the details of the case would begin to formulate themselves into a recognizable outline, the diagnosis would unravel itself, or would refuse to make itself plain, and the hunt was on. Along with that, the patient himself would shape up into something that called for attention, his peculiarities, her reticences or candors. And though I might be attracted or repelled, the professional attitude which every physician must call on would steady me, dictate the terms on which I was to proceed. Many a time a man must watch the patient's mind as it watches him, distrusting him, ready to fly off at a tangent at the first opportunity, sees himself distrusted, sees the patient turn to someone else, rejecting him.

More than once we have all seen ourselves rejected, seen some hard-pressed mother or husband go to some other adviser when we know that the advice we have given him has been correct. That too is part of the game. But in general it is the rest, the peace of mind that comes from adopting the patient's condition as one's own to be struggled with toward a solution during those few minutes or that hour or those trying days when we are searching for causes, trying to relate this to that to build a reasonable basis for action which really gives us our peace. As I say, often after I have gone into my office harassed by personal perplexities of whatever sort, fatigued physically and mentally, after two hours of intense application to the work, I came out at the finish completely rested (and I mean rested) ready to smile and to laugh as if the day were just starting.

That is why, as a writer, I have never felt that medicine interfered with me but rather that it was my very food and drink, the very thing that made it possible for me to write. Was I not interested in man? There the thing was, right in front of me. I could touch it, smell it. It was myself, naked, just as it was, without a lie telling itself to me in its own terms. Oh, I knew it wasn't for the most part giving me anything profound, but it was giving me terms, basic terms with which I could spell out matters as profound as I cared to think of.

. . . I am sure I have seen them all. And all have contributed to my pie. Let the successful carry off their blue ribbons; I have known the unsuccessful, far better persons than their more lucky brothers. One can laugh at them both, whatever the costumes they adopt. And when one is able to reveal them to themselves, high or low, they are always grateful as they are surprised that one can so have revealed their inner secrets or another's private motives. To do this is what makes a writer worth heeding: that somehow or other, whatever the source may be, he has gone to the base of the matter to lay it bare before us in terms which, try as we may, we cannot in the end escape. There is no choice then but to accept him and make him a hero.

Talking with Patients about Illness

Physicians are encouraged to believe that disease is more important than illness, and that all they need is knowledge about biology, not knowledge about the psychosocial and cultural aspects of illness.

Arthur Kleinman, MD

The first research project I completed after my fellowship was a questionnaire asking patients with chronic illness what information they needed about their illness. The topics were divided into two groups. The first group included factual medical information about the cause of the illness, the benefits and risks of medications, the role of surgery, data about long-term outcomes, self-management, and new treatments on the horizon. The second group included psychosocial issues – how to deal with the impact of the illness on the patient's personal, professional, and social life. The two types of questions were listed in random order, and patients were asked to rate the importance of each issue to them personally, and to tell us what type of healthcare professional they would like to discuss these issues with. The results of the survey were not surprising. All of the informational issues were rated highly by patients, but the psychosocial issues were consistently rated higher. And, just as important, the person whom they preferred to talk to, at least initially, for information and assistance was their doctor.

In the patient's eyes, providing guidance about the impact of the illness on their physical and emotional well-being and their roles is a critical part of their physician's job. It is something they presume we understand because we deal with illness every day. However, as they are grappling with what may be the most difficult challenge of their life, they often find that their doctor is silent about these issues. Without such counseling, people who are seriously ill are forced to "invent the wheel" on their own, stumbling through a complex maze of personal, family, and work issues. They must reorganize their life and their personal and professional goals and expectations, look for people with similar experiences from whom to get advice, and attempt to find reliable resources of information.

We know that giving attention to psychosocial issues improves outcomes. People who don't make a successful psychological adjustment to their illness are more likely to be noncompliant with treatment and less likely to return for care. In this era of unprecedented medical advances, we can't help a person who is no longer engaged or motivated to participate in their care. As Drs. Reiser and Rosen write:

> A better understanding of what the patient faces . . . is far from trivial. It is here that a physician can often make the most difference. This phase contains great opportunities for growth, increased wisdom, a greater sense of love, and enhanced spiritual meaning. It also contains an equal potential for human failure. A patient may give up, withdraw and become embittered and defeated for the rest of his life.

Unfortunately, there are significant barriers to discussion of psychosocial issues between patients and doctors. Some physicians – because of either lack of training or personality – are uncomfortable discussing emotional issues with patients, and unsure of what to say or do to offer support. Others feel that if it was not part of their training, then it is not part of their job. However, many patients have few other reliable sources of information and help, and prefer to have these conversations with a physician whom they already know and trust, and who knows them. For many people, discussing psychosocial issues with a doctor is much more acceptable than seeing a counselor or social worker, and much of the education they need about living with the particular illness requires medical knowledge that the counselor does not have.

Lack of time is an obstacle. Patients are reluctant to bring up very personal concerns when the doctor seems too busy. In the rush of daily practice, the indirect clues to a patient's distress – missed appointments, noncompliance, signs of anxiety, depression, frustration, or passivity – are unnoticed or used as an excuse: "Well, if they don't care enough to come (or take their medications), why should I?". We often don't realize that most patients don't have a clear understanding of the long-term consequences of their illness – how the damage done by an illness that goes untreated will affect their future ability to be physically, mentally, and financially independent. And if they don't understand, for whatever reason, or if life is so overwhelming that they are not focused on their health, they can't be expected to make the right decisions.

So where to begin? The complexity and diversity of each person's illness, personality, personal supports (or lack of them), finances, religion, and cultural background make the undertaking challenging. A fourth-year medical student told me about the approach of a neurologist she admired who specialized in the treatment of multiple sclerosis. "The first thing he did when he took a new patient history", she said, "was to ask the person questions about their life. Where were they from? How many children did they have? Any children still at home? What kind of work were they in? What were their hobbies?" That initial conversation allowed him to personalize the conversation later. If he did confirm the diagnosis of MS in the subsequent history and physical examination, that discussion was facilitated by the relationship he had already begun to establish. His interest in the patient as a person led them to trust him. "Patients felt like they were talking to someone who knew them and appreciated them as a person."

In medical training, we spend a lot of time drilling the "script" of the *History of Present Illness*, but there are few questions that reveal the details of the patient's life. The *Family History* is generally limited to questions about illness and death, and the *Social History* is a checklist about work, marital status, bad habits (smoking, alcohol, drugs), and sex (how often, with whom, and how). These questions, although important, are only part of the story. In the process of asking them, we divorce the disease from the illness and the patient from the person.

Atul Gawande, a surgeon and author, talks about the importance of the "unscripted question." These "off-topic" questions – about family, favorite sports teams, work, hobbies, and interests – introduce an appreciation of the person back into the encounter. And that appreciation facilitates the development of a relationship – both for the doctor and for the patient. Understanding and valuing the patient as a person lead to the empathy that motivates the physician to be to be a better communicator, educator, counselor, and advocate. And they make the patient feel that the physician respects them and their experience enough to take some extra time to get to know them. After that type of relationship has been established, people are much more likely to discuss personal issues.

INITIATING THE CONVERSATION

> All physicians are faced with the necessity of translating between the enormously complex concepts and findings of medical science and their patient's practical need to know about risk and vulnerability, disorder and treatment.
>
> Arthur Kleinman, MD

When faced with a serious illness, patients look to their physician to explain the illness, the cause, the treatment options and side-effects, the prognosis, the impact on their function in the short and long term, the time horizons in the process of care, and their role in getting better – with clarity, respect, and empathy. They are reassured and comforted when they sense that the physician has listened to them, understands who they are, and is trying to tailor the treatment for them – given their values, personal preferences, and goals. If patients understand the impact on and implications of their illness for their life, they are more likely to get involved in their care, make appropriate decisions, and to feel that they have some control over the illness.

Because conversations about the personal impact of illness often elicit emotional responses, they are more difficult than conveying medical information. People often become anxious, angry, or tearful, making the conversation more awkward both for them and for their physician. They may be surprised or

> Most practitioners . . . fall somewhere in between on this continuum which has at one end overriding concern for the science of treating disease and at the other a central interest in the art of healing illness. Effective care requires both skills, but relative inattention to the latter is particularly problematic in the care of the chronically ill.
>
> ARTHUR KLEINMAN, MD

embarrassed by the emotions that arise unexpectedly when they talk about their personal life. A friend with a chronic illness described it as follows: "When I walk into the office, I usually feel fine. I have been doing well for years. But if anyone, and I mean anyone – from the nurse, to the doctor, to the lab technician – asks me how I am doing personally, all the emotion comes rushing back and I start to cry. I feel like I have no control over it, and it's embarrassing." So, she says, she now avoids any personal discussions with her physicians.

In the face of an emotionally charged situation, there is a natural inclination – both for patients and for doctors – to look away or quickly change the subject to spare the person from embarrassment or discomfort. However, when the doctor looks or moves away, this conveys to the patient that we are uncomfortable or uninterested, or implies that the topic is inappropriate.

One of the most memorable passages from Reynolds Price's memoir about his illness was the abrupt and impersonal way in which he was given the diagnosis of a spinal cord tumor. It is an example of how to give life-changing medical information in the wrong way, in the wrong place, and at the wrong time.

> At five o'clock on that second day, I was lying on a stretcher in a crowded hallway, wearing only one of those backless hip-length gowns designed by one of the standard medical-warehouse sadists. Like all such wearers, I was passed and stared at by the usual throng of stunned pedestrians who swarm hospitals around the world.
>
> My brother Bill was standing beside me, trying as ever to lift the tone with continuous jokes – a trait of our mother's . . .
>
> I was keeping up my lifelong role, straight man to his quips, when we saw my two original doctors bound our way with a chart in hand . . .
>
> The initial internist would show his concern through years to come, but all I recall the two men saying that instant, then and there in the hallway mob scene, was "The upper ten or twelve inches of your spinal cord have swelled and are crowding the available space. The cause could be a tumor, a large cyst, or something else. We recommend immediate surgery." I could hear they were betting on a long tumor, though I'd never heard of a tumor inside the cord itself. They mentioned the name of a young staff neurosurgeon they admired, and they suggested I go back to my room and await his visit.

They moved on, leaving me and my brother empty as wind socks, stared at by strangers. . . . For now, I will flag a simple question, familiar to millions in similar corners. What would those two splendidly trained men have lost if they had waited to play their trump till I was back in a private room . . .?

At least in a private room, with the door shut, the inevitable shock of the awful news could have been absorbed, apart from the eyes of alien gawkers, by the only two human beings involved. It might have taken the doctors five minutes longer, and minutes are scarce, I understand, in their crowded days. I also understand that for doctors who work, from dawn to night, in the same drab halls, it all no doubt feels like one room. But any patient will tell them it is not, and I have often wondered how many other such devastating messages they bore that day to actual human beings unready as I for the news.

Unfortunately, we have all given life-changing information in a brusque or unsympathetic manner. We rarely mean to. Sometimes we are rushed or distracted. It might be one of hundreds of pieces of information that must be collected, analyzed, and used to make treatment decisions that day. We process so much data that we can become immune to its significance and personal impact, and then convey it with abruptness that seems insensitive to patients.

Or we make the mistake of discussing the disease as an interesting intellectual problem, as we might discuss it with colleagues, rather than as a major life-disrupting event, as the patients see it. During training and in day-to-day professional life, doctors discuss disease in terms of the pathophysiology and treatment, using technical language that facilitates and expedites the discussion, and which divorces the information from its personal implications. That type of language is perfectly appropriate for communication between physicians and healthcare providers. However, it becomes a problem when we forget to change gears in conversations with patients about illness. For patients, the disease has a very real and personal impact. For these discussions, we must not only use a different kind of language, but we also have to remember to deliver the information in a very different way – slowly, carefully, with respect, and in a private setting.

Abraham Verghese, a physician, educator, and author, wrote about the difficulty that doctors and trainees have in switching between the language they use to talk to each other and the way that they should talk to patients:

Technical language is necessary and important in diagnosis, but in such translations we might lose our ability to imagine the patient's suffering. Medical students, as they learn the voice of medicine, may begin to talk about "the diabetic foot in bed three" and "the MI in bed four." Walker Percy referred to these kinds of habits as "cowpaths", the increasingly deep ruts that we fall into whenever we take a professional language and adopt it. Any professional language brings with it the risk that it will put blinders on us, bringing about an atrophy of our imagination, a waning of the ability to understand the suffering of the patient.

After his diagnosis of cancer, Arthur Frank found that his conversations with his physicians became awkward. As a medical sociologist at an academic medical center, his doctors talked to him like a colleague rather than a person who was ill. In that professional role, he felt that he could not discuss his personal suffering with his physicians:

> We spoke over the phone as professionals: he called me Dr. Frank, I called him Dr. —. We talked about my heart as if we were talking about some computer that was producing errors in the output. . . . What was wrong with the conversation, for me as an ill person, was precisely what made the physician's performance so professional. To be professional means to be cool and management oriented. Professional talk goes this way: A problem seems to have come up, more serious than we thought, but we can still manage it. Here's our plan; any questions? Hearing this talk, I knew full well that I was being offered a deal. If my response was equally cool and professional, I would have at least a junior place on the management team . . .
>
> I did not know the cost of making that deal. . . . The demand being made of me was to treat the breakdown as if fear and frustration were not part of it, to act as if my life, my whole life, had not changed.

We all remember important conversations between doctors and patients that we observed during our training. We worked with physicians who showed unusual insight, compassion, and respect while discussing a serious diagnosis with a patient. We saw the appreciation in the eyes of the patient and their family, and left the room feeling that something important had just happened. "This is the kind of doctor I want to be", we thought, "This is why I went into medicine." However, we also witnessed interactions in which the doctor was rushed, rude, or insensitive to a patient who was feeling very vulnerable. When we left that patient's room we probably felt pretty uncomfortable – as if we were somehow complicit in giving bad care.

A fourth-year student told the following story about an unsettling interaction between a doctor and a patient. She was part of a team of physicians caring for a relatively young, single man who had had repeated surgeries for inflammatory bowel disease. "He was a cocky 'guy's guy'", she said, "You know, the kind of person who you imagine drives a beat-up pick-up truck, wears a baseball cap, and drinks a six-pack every night." But that day was different. He had been hospitalized for weeks and he was obviously and understandably discouraged. The team walked into the room to confirm the plan to proceed with a total colectomy. His gastroenterologist, a conscientious and respected physician, carefully explained the surgery, risks, and benefits.

As they walked toward the door, the patient called him back and said, awkwardly and hesitantly, that he had "just one more question." "He said that he was depressed", the student said. "He was clearly embarrassed to admit this in front of all of us. His face was flushed with emotion and you could see he was about to cry. But he was determined to get it out. It must have been very important to him." Everyone turned to the attending physician, who looked distracted and did not move back into the room or make eye contact with the patient. "There are medicines for that. I'll send someone in to talk to you", he said as he quickly turned and left the room. The student felt terrible about the interaction – so much so that she returned to the room later, on her own, to reassure the patient.

There were a number of barriers to good care and communication in that situation, including the hospital environment, the group interaction, the level of emotion in the room, and the attending physician's level of comfort and preparation for dealing with an extremely personal issue. Maybe he

> . . . the patient–physician relationship is a powerful, sometimes mysterious, frequently healing interaction between human beings. At the core of that interaction is communication. . . . A doctor's words can be gate-openers or gate-slammers: they can open the way to recovery, or they can make a patient dependent, tremulous, fearful, resistant. . . . Being able to diagnose correctly is one good test of medical competence. Being able to tell the patient what he or she has is another.
>
> NORMAN COUSINS

wanted to minimize the patient's embarrassment and thought it best to cut the conversation short. However, what he conveyed to the patient and the team was insensitivity. His inability to reassure the patient that their reaction to the stress of the illness was very normal and that he was there to help increased the patient's sense of failure, weakness, and isolation.

Given the importance of these discussions to patients and to the relationship between doctors and patients, how should you discuss psychosocial issues with patients? Most of us learn what to say by observing doctor–patient interactions during training, or by thinking about how we would like to be treated if we were ill. However, that type of learning can be haphazard and incomplete. There are ways to make these conversations easier and more productive. Whether you are talking to patients about critical medical issues or psychosocial issues, here are some strategies to facilitate a difficult conversation.

- Hold the conversation in the right setting. In the hospital, try to find a quiet room where disruptions will be minimized. Turn your pager off. In the office, you can schedule the patient for the end of the day, when you have more time. If an issue comes up unexpectedly, during a busy day, listen, offer support, and then consider asking the patient to return for a follow-up appointment so the two of you will have more uninterrupted time to discuss it properly.

  You might say:
  - *I think this issue is very important and the two of us are going to need some time to discuss it. How would you feel about coming in on Friday and I will block out some time for us to talk. Meanwhile, you and I can both think about resources that might be helpful.*

- Sit down. Don't conduct important conversations while standing looking down at a patient lying in bed or sitting in a chair. Eye-to-eye conversations put you and the patient at the same level, as equals in the discussion. When you take a minute to sit down, you let the patient know that you recognize the importance of the issue and that you are willing to take the time needed to discuss it.

- Learn to listen well and with full attention. Let the patient tell their story, at least initially, without interruption. This conveys respect and shows your interest.

↪ If multiple physicians or trainees are present, decide who will do the talking, and remind the others to listen quietly and not to come and go from the room.

↪ Include the patient in every discussion at bedside or office teaching rounds, asking them if they will allow you to go over the history, exam, and test results with the trainees. This allows the patient to be a teacher with you, rather than the object of an intellectual discussion they may or may not understand.

↪ Maintain eye contact during a difficult conversation, even if the patient is angry or tearful. Looking away suggests that you are uncomfortable or, worse, disinterested, and discourages the patient from continuing.

↪ Learn to be comfortable with silence. Sitting quietly with a patient who is tearful, angry, or depressed creates a moment of calm and time in which to process what has been said. Avoid the tendency to offer a quick or pat solution to move the conversation on. Acknowledge the patient's frustration, fear, isolation, sorrow, grief, or loss, and the magnitude of the impact of the illness on their life.

> I always assumed that if I became seriously ill, physicians, no matter how overworked, would somehow recognize what I was living through. I did not know what form it would take, but I assumed it would happen. What I experienced was the opposite. The more critical my diagnosis became, the more reluctant physicians were to talk to me. I had difficulty getting them to make eye contact; most came only to see my disease.
>
> ―――――――――――
> ARTHUR FRANK, MD

You might say:
- *I am so sorry that you have to go through this.*
- *It sounds like it has been a very lonely time for you.*
- *It must be very difficult to go though this illness feeling that no one really understands what is happening to you.*

↪ Allow people time to mourn their losses. After a diagnosis of a serious illness, doctors are focused on moving forward and the treatment of disease. However, many patients need time to discuss and understand their illness and its impact on their life, and are not ready to move on to treatment.

⌒ Look for signs of depression, anxiety, denial, and hopelessness – noncompliance with medication, missed visits, poor eye contact, weight loss, or the patient who seems totally uninvolved in their care.

⌒ Recognize, discuss, and respond to angry patients. Patients under stress respond in a variety of ways. If they are angry about their vulnerability and lack of control they may direct that anger at the most vulnerable physicians – the students and trainees. It may be something subtle – a patient who makes comments about your personal appearance or asks personal questions that make you feel uncomfortable – or a more blatant verbal attack. Feeling embarrassed, confused, and perhaps a bit guilty ("I must have done something wrong to cause this reaction"), students and residents often say nothing about difficult interactions with patients. Medical training is a kind of endurance test, and students and residents often assume that this is just one more unpleasant part of medical training that they have to put up with. The "code of silence" in medicine reinforces this assumption – there are many unpleasant things that are never discussed. However, if you feel threatened by a patient (either verbally or physically) or uncomfortable, you should excuse yourself and discuss the issue with a colleague, the staff, or a senior physician. Talking about these encounters forces the team to recognize a problem that they may have ignored and, just as important, may protect other people involved in the patient's care.

Recognize your own emotional reactions to patients. Don't take anger personally – anger and criticism may be a sign of the patient's feelings of guilt, fear, or anxiety, or a reaction to the indignity caused by illness and medical care. And don't respond to a patient with anger. If you feel yourself becoming angry, try to sit quietly, nod, listen, and acknowledge the anger – even if you feel that you are not responsible for the problems.

You might say:

⌒ *I am sorry this happened to you, Mr. —. I will talk with the doctors and nurses involved in your care and see if we can figure this out.*

Or, simply:

— *Is there anything I can do to help?*

If there are delays, miscommunications, complications, or errors, discuss them with the patient and offer an apology. Doctors are often afraid to say they are sorry when the process of medical care has been difficult or imperfect, whether or not it is their fault. They may be worried litigation could have a significant personal and financial impact on their career. However, studies show that a personal conversation and apology can diffuse blame and confrontation

When patients are ill, dealing with the medical bureaucracy can be overwhelming. Patients and their families often feel that they are cogs in an impersonal machine that has no understanding of their suffering, and they are much more likely to get angry with impersonal systems when things go wrong. Taking time to sit down with a patient and/ or their family establishes a personal relationship, demonstrates your respect for them, their situation, and their feelings, and decreases the likelihood of confrontation and litigation.

WHAT TO SAY

> Talking to doctors always makes me conscious of what I am not supposed to say. Thus I am particularly silent when I am given bad news. I know I am only supposed to ask about the disease, but what I feel is the illness. The questions I want to ask about my life are not allowed, not speakable, not even thinkable. The gap between what I feel and what I feel allowed to say widens and deepens and swallows my voice.
>
> *Arthur Frank, MD*

Educate

When faced with a serious, life-threatening, or disabling disease or disorder, patients look to their physician to diagnose and treat and, just as important, to educate them about the course of the disease and to prepare them for its impact on their life and their role in getting better. Generally, we are good at the first two, but not always so good at the last. As we move from room to room, evaluating problems and quickly making treatment decisions, we often forget that if the patient doesn't see what we see (the long-term damage that occurs without treatment) or understand what we understand (how and when treatments work, how responses will be monitored, etc.), they can't make the appropriate decisions.

> What the patient cannot put into words, the physician must understand. What the patient won't put into words, the physician must speak for him. He must hear the words the patient doesn't say and be sensitive to the anguish that cannot be expressed. . . . This is compassion.
>
> PHILIP TUMULTY, PHD

The word "doctor" is derived from the Latin word for "educator." Among physicians, pediatricians really understand this role best. They educate parents using a technique called "anticipatory guidance." At each routine visit, they discuss the developmental issues that are likely to arise, and offer strategies for dealing with them in advance. All types of physicians, from primary care to specialists, can use the same technique to help patients with critical illnesses to anticipate the physical and personal challenges that lie ahead.

Many patients are relatively young and immature when they are first diagnosed with an illness, and even the most mature patient may have a very limited understanding of the potential impact of a serious illness on their life. The average person with a chronic illness spends less time in a year with their doctor then they spend buying shoes. However, the decisions that they make between those visits will have a profound effect on their longevity and quality of life. How do we adequately prepare to make those decisions?

It is the physician's job to "paint a picture" of what is happening, what the future holds, and how the patient can influence the outcome. Over the initial visits, the goal is to help the patient to understand the diagnosis, treatment alternatives, toxicities, and time line of care – the "ifs" and "thens." Since most people are visual learners, sketches, diagrams, pictures, and handouts are more effective in communicating the basic information clearly and simply. Patients are more compliant with medications and make better decisions about how to use them when they have an understanding of how they work, when they work, how we know that they are working, and their side-effects. Patients who are given a new diagnosis should always be provided with written material or, if they have access to the Internet, electronic sources of information.

The progression of some diseases – whether it be loss of heart, kidney, liver, or lung function – is often asymptomatic in the early stages, and therefore invisible to patients. If they forget to take their medication and notice no change in how they feel, they may make poor decisions about compliance. By explaining how their response to treatment will be measured and sharing the results of those outcome measures – X-rays, laboratory tests, or physical exam findings – over time, you reinforce compliance. If the results are visible – on a computer screen or printout – they will have more impact.

Graph out and give patients the results of their tests over time, relating them to the medications and treatments. Encourage the patient to ask questions, and ask them to tell you what they understand about the illness or treatment. Patients who are engaged in their care are more likely to take their medication and return for treatment.

Paint a picture of the long-term aspects of the disease that will help patients to weigh the risks and benefits of treatment, and give them the information that they will need to plan their professional and personal life. We sometimes keep the long-term aspects of illness to ourselves in order to protect patients, because it is uncertain, or because we are rushed. However, people need to understand not only where the illness is today, but also where it is likely to go.

For example, a woman with rheumatoid arthritis told me that she was very reluctant to take disease-modifying drugs after her diagnosis. Her pain from arthritis was not that great, and she was concerned about the infection risks and unknown long-term consequences of new therapies. Ten years later, after she had sustained significant damage to her shoulders and wrists, she was at a medical conference where she heard a speaker discuss how those treatments might not only have had a profound impact on her mobility and function, but also lessened the risk of heart attack and stroke:

> She said, "When I was diagnosed, my doctor told me that I should take these drugs so I would have less pain and less joint inflammation and damage. But he never explained that there was a time after which the damage was done and the treatments would not be effective. If he had told me that I could

lose my physical independence and would be at higher risk for strokes and heart attacks, I would have decided differently".

Explain the likely impact of the disease and treatments, in the various stages, on physical function – at work and at home – and on mood. Over the first few visits, get a sense of what the patient's daily activities and responsibilities are. Try to give some time line with regard to what to expect in the future – how likely the treatment is to work, how long it will take to know whether it is working, when and if the patient will return to work, the pros and cons of leaving work and applying for disability benefits, and the options that are available if the initial treatment does not work. Think about what information you would want to be given if you were faced with a similar illness. This information can be shared over a number of visits, and repeated and reinforced over time.

Ask about psychosocial issues

By asking about psychosocial issues – about mood, sleep, family, and work – you acknowledge that these are a typical part of the adjustment to illness (especially when there are recurrent setbacks or complications, or the outcome is unclear for some time). Just knowing that their reactions are normal and not a sign of their own weakness is reassuring to patients. By raising these issues, you signal your willingness to talk about them. No matter how worried they are, many patients will not raise these issues unless you ask.

Even if you have no immediate answer or way to decrease their distress, you can reassure the patient that changes in mood often improve with time, and that it may take a sustained period of "calm" before they will feel less anxious and fearful.

For example, you might say:

⌒ *Many of the people with this illness feel overwhelmed at times or feel anxious or depressed. It is a very normal part of going through such a difficult experience as this. Have you felt this way?*

⌒ *I know that living with this illness is difficult and stressful. How are you doing? Are you getting the support you need?*

⌒ *How is your family handling your illness? Do you think they understand what is happening? Are they supportive?*

⌒ *How are things at work? Have you talked to people about your illness? What was their reaction?*

Discuss the importance of maintaining personal relationships with family and friends

Illness is isolating, and relationships are frequently strained. Reactions of friends, family, and co-workers to serious illness are difficult to predict. Some people are uncomfortable with illness, and others just don't understand the seriousness of the illness or its impact on the patient. Remind the patient that friends who seem to avoid them, or avoid discussing their illness, may simply not know what to say or how to say it. Others will overreact, taking over where they are not needed, or offering advice or information that is not helpful. Human relationships are imperfect, but the vulnerability of illness can intensify the normal feeling of disappointment and being let down when friends and family do not offer appropriate help.

Encourage patients to re-establish a daily routine

During periods of disability that take people away from their usual activities, time spent alone at home can increase isolation, worry, and anxiety. Home can begin to feel like a prison where there is too much time to think. Everyone else comes and goes, telling stories at the end of the day about what they've done and who they've met, but the patient has no stories to tell. People need a focus and a purpose to the day – a reason to get up in the morning. Talk about the importance of finding activities that help to pass the time, that distract them from worry, and that if possible get them out of the house.

Encourage regular physical activity

Exercise improves sleep, decreases anxiety, and improves long-term outcomes in most illnesses. Ted Kooser and Arthur Frank found that their daily walk was an integral part of their physical and emotional recovery. The routine of exercise gives a focus to the day, peaceful time for thinking and planning, and a way to achieve some control over the illness. Exercise can improve endurance and appearance and increase self-esteem.

> Physicians often do not express to the patient that they recognize their experience of fear, frustration, and personal change. . . . But physicians' self-imposed limitations dictate the reciprocal roles patients are expected to play. . . . All illness (particularly AIDS) has two dimensions: a physical deficit and a spiritual violation. And when there is no cure, the one thing we can offer is to really understand the story that is playing out, to aid and abet its satisfactory conclusion.
>
> ABRAHAM VERGHESE, MD

Motivating patients to exercise is extraordinarily challenging. Their energy levels are likely to be low. They may feel anxious, depressed, unmotivated, or overwhelmed by their family and work responsibilities. Some patients are unwilling or unable to leave the house. In these situations, a supervised home program of physical therapy can be very helpful. Regular contact with a health professional such as a physical therapist, nurse, or counselor – who listens, reassures, cajoles, gossips, and laughs with them – improves motivation and provides emotional support that can decrease anxiety and depression. These professionals also provide very helpful information about what is going on in the home, which gives the doctor a much broader view of how the patient is functioning and what supports are available.

Acknowledge in advance that medical care is frustrating and imperfect

The bureaucracy of medical care is impersonal and difficult to deal with when one is ill. Admit that some of the healthcare professionals involved in the patient's care will not always be understanding or empathetic. Inevitably miscommunications, mishaps, cancellations, delays, and mistakes will occur. It might be something as small as a lab order that is not available when they come to clinic, a last-minute cancellation of a long-awaited appointment, or something as important as a serious side-effect of treatment. Offer to be their advocate to smooth what is almost always a frustrating experience and sometimes a humiliating one.

Best of all, with the help of friends, I managed to laugh a few times most days. Sometimes the out-of-practice chuckle reminded me of how a gift as big as the tendency to laugh in the face of disaster is a literally biochemical endowment.

REYNOLDS PRICE

Humor

Find ways to laugh with your patients when this is possible. Humor is a constructive way to deal with the frustrations, indignities, and ironies of medical care and illness, and allows the patient to rise above them, if only for a moment. Appropriate shared humor and laughter diffuse anger, relieve anxiety, diminish pain, and help people to see a situation from a different perspective.

Distractions

For many people who are seriously ill, the

illness becomes all they can think about. Finding distractions that can take their mind away from that worry is challenging. A 35-year-old writer and father of three told me about the importance of music during his recovery from cancer. He spent extended periods of time at home alone during his treatment. Although he was an avid reader, after his diagnosis he found that he couldn't concentrate long enough to read. He couldn't watch TV because sad endings upset him. He couldn't listen to the radio because bad news was unsettling and made him more anxious. But, he could listen to music.

So he recorded music from different periods of his life on his iPod – music from the summer he had his first girlfriend, music played by his high school and college bands, and music from the first dance with his wife. He chose songs that reminded him of people and places he had known, and things he had done – pieces that he thought were beautiful, peaceful, or outrageous. He played this music during chemotherapy, radiation therapy, while he was waiting in the lab or office, or when he was at home alone feeling anxious or in low spirits. His friends and children recorded music to keep him company and remind him of them when he was alone. Music kept him in touch with life, the person he had been, and the people who were important to him during the most discouraging and vulnerable parts of his treatment.

Communicate your respect for the patient's fortitude, courage, and persistence

Low self-esteem is part and parcel of life with illness. Sometimes people just feel whipped – that they are not the funny, brave, thoughtful, or patient person they hoped they would be. They are sure that if they were a better person, they would handle the illness better. The reassurance and respect of their physician, who may be the only person who understands the ordeal they are living through, can be tremendously supportive to patients. Remind the patient that sometimes the best anyone can do is to get through the illness one day at a time.

You might say:

- *This has been a difficult time for you, and I know that sometimes you think that you should handle the stress of this illness better. But I think that you have handled it remarkably well. You have moved ahead with courage and determination. I know you have felt overwhelmed and emotionally exhausted – that sometimes you feel like you can't face another day. But you keep going day after day, one foot in front of the other. Sometimes that is all you can do – keep going. I have tremendous respect for you and the courage you have shown in living with this illness.*

Recognize pain and suffering

Sometime during the busy hospital day, take the time to go back to see a patient who is struggling with a difficult illness. Sit down and, looking directly at them, discuss the new information that has come from the tests and consulting physicians, outline the plans for the next few days, and answer their questions. Let them know that you realize what an overwhelming experience the illness and hospitalization have been.

You might say:
- *I know this is a very difficult time for you. Please let me know if there is anything I can do.*

You can do the same thing at the end of an office visit, taking a few extra minutes to tell patients you recognize the difficulty of living with the illness.

Try to alleviate feelings of guilt and anger

Many patients have second thoughts about what they or someone else could or should have done that might have prevented the illness or improved the outcome. The notion that some or all of the pain that they and their family are living with could have been prevented can haunt people for years. We all look for a reason why life-altering events happen in our lives, and that search can lead to blame. Allow people time to discuss their guilt and anger, help them to put them into perspective, and then encourage them to move on.

Counseling

If a patient is very anxious, depressed, or isolated, counseling can be very helpful. Many people do not want to repeatedly burden family or friends with their anxieties and worries. Relationships become unbalanced when you are the one always asking for support. Counseling and support groups offer patients a place to speak openly and honestly about their adjustment to illness, work out strategies to deal with their problems, and obtain independent feedback about their reactions. The physician can point out the value of these services and reassure patients that counseling is a constructive and proactive way to deal with significant stress – and not something that they should feel is stigmatizing or a sign of personal weakness.

Emphasize privacy

Medical information is private. Once it is out, it can't be taken back. Let patients know upfront that friends, colleagues, and complete strangers who become aware of a person's illness often offer unwanted and/or incorrect information that can be distressing, despite their best intentions to be helpful. Decisions about sharing information with friends, employees, and co-workers should be made carefully and thoughtfully.

Medication for sleep and mood

The diagnosis of a serious illness, like other overwhelming life stresses, is often accompanied by periods of insomnia. People find their thoughts racing late into the night as they try to take it all in and plan. Anxiety and depression also interfere with sleep. And everything seems worse – more hopeless, depressing, and discouraging – in the middle of the night. Short-term insomnia is treatable, but we almost never ask about it and so it often goes untreated. A prescription for sleep medication or medication to manage anxiety can be very helpful, especially in the first few weeks after diagnosis or after major setbacks.

> Physicians and nurses often forget that when treatment runs out, there can still be care. Simply recognizing suffering for what it is, regardless of whether it can be treated, is care.
>
> _____
>
> ARTHUR FRANK, MD

Persistent anxiety and depression are common problems in serious and chronic illness. As the months go by, remember to ask about mood and to treat anxiety and depression with medication when appropriate. Recognize your limitations in the use of these medications, and rely on consultants when these problems are unresponsive to your attempts at treatment.

Express concern and support

When there is no medical treatment left and you are unable to come up with a "solution", remember the importance of expressing your concern and your willingness to advocate for a patient's needs.

Try to leave patients with realistic hope, and recognize those who have lost hope

When patients seem to be losing hope, ask about the broader social situation. What is happening in the family? What is happening to their relationships?

Do they have a support structure? Are there financial problems? Involve other members of the healthcare team – the chaplains, social workers, physical therapists, and nurses – and talk with the patient's family and significant others.

> For many who cannot see hope, their vision is blurred because they believe that they are unable to exert any level of control over their circumstances. When I discover such patients . . . I try to discover why they feel so completely at the mercy of the forces around them.
>
> I learned that it takes much more than mere words to communicate information and alter affect. . . . I try to let patients read in my eyes that there is true hope for them. . . . Even then, the stated facts and the chance of prevailing are often best articulated in more than one voice. Doctors are fallible, not only in how they wield a scalpel or prescribe a drug, but in the language they use. Family and friends, clergy and social workers, psychologists and counselors, and, often most compelling, other patients . . . can better speak from personal experience and reach the roots of despair and distrust.
>
> *Jerome Groopman, MD*

The Impact of Illness on the Family

Chronic illness is like an uninvited guest who arrives on your doorstep with all his baggage and invades everyone's space. Each member of the family is affected psychologically by this guest, and while it is clear that he is staying for the duration, no one knows exactly why he has come, and what will happen while he is here.

Linda Welsh

You walk into her hospital room at 2 a.m. in the morning, the last of three people – the intern, the resident, and now you, the third-year student – to perform the same history and physical examination on Mrs. Roberts. An attractive woman with wavy rich brown hair and fair, almost translucent skin, she is clearly exhausted, but sits attentively in bed answering all your questions. You will be in and out quickly, you think. You'll get the write-up done and go home.

Mrs. Roberts has chronic leukemia and she is admitted for a cough and fever. "Pneumonia", her doctors told her, and "chronic anemia." You glance through your list of questions and then get to the family history. She has three children and her husband works in construction, she says. You quickly finish your exam, so that you both can get some sleep. You thank her and get up to leave.

"I am exhausted", you hear her say as you reach the door. You look back into the dimly lit room and see her sitting in bed, head down, starting to cry, and looking defeated.

"My husband and children, they just don't understand." You go back and stand by her bed, feeling unprepared and inadequate, not knowing what to say. So you tell her that she will be better after the transfusion, some sleep, and when the pneumonia is treated. But she looks desolate, un-consoled, and alone. She goes on to tell you that her husband doesn't really understand the seriousness of her illness, and that they never discuss it. She has young children who need care and a teenage daughter who is being rebellious. "Everyone tells me that I look fine. No one helps."

Patients often reveal their fears and worries to the unassuming medical student or intern who wanders into their quiet hospital room in the middle of the night. These conversations begin our education about the profound effects of illness on the family and on family dynamics. You wonder why no one was helping, what it is like to be the teenage child of a mother who is chronically ill and, most important, what you can possibly say to help.

The impact of serious illness on the family can be devastating. The changes in roles and family dynamics are one of the most difficult challenges for patients, but it can be equally difficult for the partner and for the children. How much should a parent or partner say about the illness or expect from those around them? When is it time to give up some of their responsibilities and who should they ask for help? How do they ask for help? How should they handle strained relationships with their partner or children?

Parents doggedly hold on to their roles and relationships with their children. For many, this is the role that they treasure most and are least likely to give up or allow to change. Because of unrealistic expectations about what they can do – cleaning the house, maintaining the yard, driving the car pools, cooking, coaching – they don't ask for the help they need, hoping that maybe, with time, things will get better. Their instinct is to protect the family from the impact of illness. To accomplish this, they may keep them at arm's length, never fully informing their partner or children about their diagnosis, prognosis, or the impact of the treatment. Often they can't adequately prepare their family because they don't have a full understanding of the illness, the treatments, or how their life is about to change.

Denial, disability, anxiety, and depression can all prevent an ill parent or their stressed partner from reorganizing family roles and responsibilities and getting appropriate help so that the needs of the children and the household are met. Single parents may have no one available to help. When the illness worsens or goes through periods of exacerbation, lack of planning precipitates periods of crisis because there is no plan in place for friends or family members to fill in. The person who is ill can feel profound disappointment when they don't get the support they need from family or friends, even though they may never have told them what they need.

The relationships between couples – their roles and responsibilities – change during a serious illness, sometimes temporarily but often permanently. The life and goals of the partner are dramatically and sometimes abruptly altered, without warning or a period of planning and adjustment. Who is the caretaker? Who is the breadwinner? Who is maintaining the household? Who is understanding and meeting the needs of the children?

Physical and sexual relationships change. Both partners may be exhausted by the combination of the time demands of treatment and the unchanged needs of their work and family. Overwhelmed by fatigue and worry, they may only have the energy to meet basic family needs and then have time to rest. Feeling that they have become a burden, the person who is ill is reluctant to discuss the illness, but may find that they have little else to say. The healthy partner feels too guilty to complain about the negative impact of the illness on them, and an uncomfortable silence ensues. Each feels isolated and unsupported, and they may retreat into opposite corners for months or years to come.

As discouraging as this sounds, with time most couples eventually find a new equilibrium and adjust to their different expectations. As they move through the diagnostic testing and treatment together, they share an intense period of vulnerability and uncertainty. Through this new intimacy and the caretaking that the illness demands, they may find that their relationship is renewed and reinforced. Unfortunately, for some this highly stressful period exacerbates pre-existing tensions and problems with commitment to the relationship that are insurmountable.

ILLNESS AND RELATIONSHIPS WITH CHILDREN

The child of a parent who is seriously ill is often confused about the cause and severity of the illness and their role in helping. During periods when the parent is absent from the home, or is at home but disabled, children may feel worried and unsettled by the change in routine, or abandoned by a parent who is physically or emotionally unable to care for them. Very young children often float through a parent's illness, oblivious to what is happening. They are more flexible in accepting the changed dynamics in the family so long as someone is meeting their needs. However, whether or not they are old enough to understand the illness itself, the changed family dynamics are usually stressful.

Because they are at a time in life when they are most self-absorbed, pre-adolescent and adolescent children have the most difficult time adjusting to an illness in the family. Some are disappointed to have a parent who is unable to meet their needs at home, or to fulfill their social functions in the community, or who doesn't look and act like other parents. A few will overcompensate by becoming caretakers. Others feel guilty that they should be doing more to help, but don't know what to do or don't want that role or responsibility. They may secretly wish for a parent who is more like other parents, and spend as much time away from them as possible in order to avoid having to deal with the illness or the strained relationships in the family. And so they may start to feel guilty about their desire to be like every other teenager.

In families where there is severe illness, children can fade into the background as their parents are consumed by the financial and physical impact of the illness and are less aware of the child's thoughts, worries, or fears. Adolescents are at high risk of taking advantage of the lack of attention and supervision by engaging in risky behaviors. Stressed or lonely teenagers may look to the wrong people for escape or companionship.

Alliances between children and parents change when a parent has a psychologically or physically disabling illness. Children begin to look to the parent who is well or to people outside the family to meet their needs. And these individuals are likely to have a different approach to roles and responsibilities and a different way of prioritizing what needs to be done. New tensions between the parents or between parents and children may arise. All of these changes require time for adjustment.

Most partners and children are very helpful and attentive in the initial stages of a serious illness but, if the illness is chronic, this attention may fade. If the parent looks well, the children and partner may not understand the impact of the illness on their energy or stamina, and unrealistically expect that they will resume their old roles and responsibilities.

What can the physician do about all of this? Again, use anticipatory guidance. Mention to the patient that illness and disability often bring changes in family dynamics. Through conversations spread over multiple visits, you can help the patient to develop a realistic understanding of the impact of the illness and its treatment on their ability to function and their roles in the family. That understanding allows them to make appropriate plans. Some issues to discuss are listed below.

Information and Communication

Encourage the patient to share information with their family. Remind them that it is important that their partner has a full understanding of the course and physical impact of the illness and treatment. Together they should decide how to give basic information to the children about the illness, as appropriate for each child's age. Lack of information may cause more worry than appropriate information, and also means that the partner and the children have no constructive way to help.

Invite the patient to bring their partner, family members, or older children to an office visit. Including them in the visit gives them a chance to understand the illness, the treatment, the prognosis, and the impact of the illness on day-to-day function. At these visits, you can validate the patient's symptoms to a partner or family member who is not sympathetic or not offering appropriate support. You can also reassure a family member who is overly protective or alarmist that the patient is getting well and can do more. It is an opportunity to talk about family dynamics, the effect of illness on children and their reactions to the ill parent, and enables the patient and their partner to make concrete plans as to how each family member or friend can help. Most people want to help and to offer support, but just don't know what to say or how to do it.

Planning

Encourage the patient to make realistic plans to get the support they need. By giving their partner, children and friends jobs, they help them to find a role and allow them to be involved. If they are too ill to do this, their partner or a family member may be willing to take on this role. These tasks give friends and family a sense of accomplishment and lessen guilt and anxiety. Just as important, they make the patient feel cared for.

Set Priorities

Advise the patient to set priorities. If they can't do everything, then it is time to let the less important things go. For example, an orderly and perfectly clean home is not essential, nor is complete control over their children's diets, bedtime, room cleanliness, and attire. They should save their time for and invest their emotional energy in their relationships, keeping the household functioning and their spirits up. Years from now, their children will not remember how clean the house was, how well the lawn was maintained, or who made the food, but they will remember time spent with their parents. Being an exhausted parent with an organized house is less important than being a rested parent who has time to listen, laugh, notice, and participate.

Community Resources

Referral to patient support groups is very helpful for families during the initial period of diagnosis and treatment, when they are stunned and trying to understand what is happening. Books, patient education material, and face-to-face meetings with other people who are dealing with illness can help families to learn strategies for coping and feel less isolated. Information and guidance about referrals to local social service agencies, including disability, home health aids, visiting nurses, and vocational rehabilitation counseling, provides additional supports to the family.

Counseling

Reassure the patient that their partner and children can benefit from counseling to help them to adjust to the new family dynamics and responsibilities. A referral of a child, partner, or family for medication or counseling is not a sign of their family's failure or weakness. Rather, it is an appropriate way to respond to the significant life change caused by a serious or disabling illness. Develop a list of resources such as support groups, voluntary health associations, community groups, and psychiatrists and counselors who specialize in the psychosocial impact of illness on people. If this list is easily available, you will find that you use it over and over again.

Involvement with Advocacy Groups

Over time, many patients, partners, and children feel energized and find direction through their work with patient advocacy groups. The "Walks" and events that these groups sponsor are a way for families and friends to turn out and show support in a fun, less sober environment. Children have an opportunity to see other families who are affected by illness. Some families find hope and meaning in illness by becoming active advocates at a regional and national level.

Time

Adjustment to a new family dynamic will inevitably take time. All the educating, planning, and counseling won't change the reality that life is not what was expected or planned for. Despite everyone's best intentions, people will be impatient, get angry, act out, or feel isolated. The game pieces on the chessboard have been toppled, and it will take some time to reorganize everyone's place and roles.

As a physician, the simplest and most important thing you can do, over months to years of care, is to continue to ask how the family is doing. Family dynamics may be stable for years at a time, but new stresses are bound to arise – the partner who appeared to be supportive for years abruptly leaves or becomes ill, there are financial problems, or a child is having difficulties. These changes in support bring back the vulnerability and uncertainty that can exacerbate anxiety and depression. The lives of people with serious illness are susceptible to the same changes that we all face, but their dependence on the support of the people around them makes the impact of those changes greater. Just listening is helpful.

Advocacy

. . . the primary physician on a case is not only the care provider but should also assume the role of patient advocate. I now take this role more seriously than ever.

. . . I have become more outspoken in this regard as well. . . . In the past I would have been more reticent about such things, but if the physician in charge doesn't stick up for his patients, then who will?

Charles Kleinman, MD

In the increasingly complex world of medical diagnosis and treatment, the care we provide for patients often cannot be contained in an office visit. More and more patients need an advocate to help them to navigate what can be an unwieldy and sometimes unsympathetic system, making calls to insurers to authorize treatments and to collaborating healthcare providers to coordinate care and improve communication. The mark of a truly outstanding physician is his or her willingness to take the time to contact other providers to review the medical and personal history of a seriously ill patient and forward all of the information necessary to expedite their care. These calls can be time consuming (taken out of a day in which there is rarely extra time) and the time taken is rarely reimbursed. However, advocacy is of great value to patients, especially early in an illness when they may feel overwhelmed and less able to be confident and assertive.

Physicians are often accused of having a "silo" attitude towards healthcare, in that they are only aware of what happens in the hospital and office. However, the outcome of illness and the effectiveness of treatment are often determined by what happens in the home and the community. Directing patients to people and resources that will help them to live with illness and disability – patient advocacy groups, social services, resources to help with the cost of medication, and other health professionals – is equally important during recovery.

Beyond this individual advocacy, there is advocacy to improve the efficiency, quality, and responsiveness of healthcare for all patients. This might involve work with local patient groups, voluntary health associations, or political advocacy groups at a state or national level. The personal and time demands of an average medical practice make this level of involvement seem daunting. However, it can be accomplished over a career and through the support of groups that advocate for improvements in healthcare.

> Responsibility for the care of patients cannot end with the care of individuals. Each of us who participates in this endeavor also bears some responsibility for sustaining and improving a system of care so that it regularly and readily provides optimal care. How can it be done? In my experience, it has required some unexpected endeavors.
>
> JOANNE LYNNE, *EMPATHY AND THE PRACTICE OF MEDICINE*

Association of American Medical Colleges (AAMC), 1998
Physicians must be dutiful:

Physicians must feel obliged to collaborate with other health professionals and to use systematic approaches for promoting, maintaining, and improving the health of individuals and populations. They must understand how to utilize disease- and injury-prevention practices in the care of individuals and their families, and in public education practices in their communities, and must be advocates for improving access to care for everyone, especially those members of the traditionally underserved populations. They must understand the economic, psychological, occupational, social, and psychological factors that contribute to the development or perpetration of conditions that impair health. In caring for individual patients, they must apply the principles of evidence-based medicine and cost-effectiveness in making decisions about utilization of limited resources. They must be committed to working collaboratively with other physicians, other healthcare professionals (including administrators of hospitals, healthcare organizations, and systems of care), and individuals representing a wide variety of community agencies. As members of a team addressing individual or population-based healthcare issues, they must be willing to provide leadership when appropriate, and defer to the leadership of others when indicated. They must acknowledge and respect the roles of other healthcare professionals in providing needed services to individual patients, populations, or communities.

Report 1: Learning Objectives for Medical Student
Education – Guidelines for Medical Schools.

SECTION 3

Reflections of Doctors on Illness, Medical Training, and Clinical Care

As I started to think seriously about telling my story, other aspects of my experience came to mind. Sooner or later all doctors become patients, a role change that is never easy, although it does provide insights that are not learned in medical school. My time came sooner, it came early in my career and, strangely, in my own hands – I made my own diagnosis. In the aftermath of my diagnosis I learned a great deal that is not to be found in medical textbooks. My experience made me both a greater admirer and a harsher critic of my profession, and intensified my desire to describe what happened for the benefit of doctors and patients.

Fitzhugh Mullan, MD

It is 8 a.m. on a morning in early May, and I look up from the podium and survey the auditorium that is still dimly lit and relatively empty. There are clusters of second-year medical students scattered in the seats – some in small groups talking and laughing, some sitting alone sipping coffee or sleeping. Over the next 20 minutes, as I talk, a few more students wander quietly down the aisles. Although they are usually good humored, almost all of them have that glazed "hit me again" look as they gear up for a discussion of another of over a hundred diseases they have been trying to cram into their memory this year.

As I begin the lecture before clinic, I do something slightly manipulative. I start by saying "Rheumatoid arthritis can be a devastating chronic illness, affecting 1 in 100 people, and one of those people could be you." Why do I say this? Partly it is my way of trying to grab their attention as they sit there half asleep – and a few heads do look up, slightly startled. However, it is also a way to nudge them into imagining, as I progress through the discussion, "What if that was me?"

When I give the weekly morning lecture to a group of four to six third-year medical students and residents before clinic, I do essentially the same thing. As I describe the different treatments for a condition – say lupus – I look around the table, point to them one at a time, and say "OK, let's say that you have lupus with kidney involvement, and you have arthritis, and you have severe skin disease, and you're three months pregnant (pointing to one of the male students). How would your treatments differ?" And I notice that they look a little more engaged, and sometimes slightly uncomfortable. What I am trying to do is to help them cross the line, in their imagination, from doctor to patient, and to remind them, as Fitzhugh Mullan says, that we all become patients sooner or later – that the people they will be treating are people like them, and that any of us could have our lives changed by serious illness at any time. Does my approach have a lasting effect? Probably not, but it does pose a question that I hope they will continue to consider as they care for people through their training.

In this book, the experience of illness has been explored largely through the writings of physicians. It is easier for people to empathize with someone they can identify with, and this is no different for doctors. However, just as important, physicians' training and experience in medicine give them important insights into what works and what doesn't work in modern medical care, and they express it in a way that other doctors can relate to. They have had the opportunity to clearly view medical care from "both sides of the bedrail."

This book begins with a description of the personal impact of illness using first-hand narratives, and then goes on to discuss the important role of the doctors in offering advice and guidance to the people for whom they care about how to live with illness. This last section includes excerpts from the essays of physicians about their own illness. In their own words, they tell us how illness changed the way they view medical care, the way they practice medicine, and the way they treat patients.

What they say is not surprising. Most write that their illness helped them to understand the personal impact of fear, vulnerability, and loss of control in a way that their medical education and practice had not. Frequently, they talk about their disappointment with the impersonal medical bureaucracy, the indignities of medical care, and the lack of empathy shown by their physicians and other healthcare providers. Living through an illness that was, for most of them, the most difficult experience of their life helped them to be more understanding with their own patients and more willing to take time with them and offer them support. Their experience clarified the importance of empathy, education, communication, psychosocial support, and advocacy in patient care, and changed their attitudes to the practice of medicine.

Fitzhugh Mullan, MD is an academic internist. As a young physician, he diagnosed his own cancer, seminoma, for which he received radiation and surgery. There were significant complications, including infections that required disfiguring surgery and prolonged hospitalizations. He wrote a book, *Vital Signs, A Young Doctor's Struggle with Cancer*, about the personal impact of the illness on him, his family, and his work.

> So what have I learned from the experience of cancer? I have learned what it is like to be a hospital patient, learned how vitally important nursing staff

are to patient morale. For my 48 hours postop, I was completely helpless and totally dependent on the nursing staff to keep me in one piece. I shall be eternally grateful to those nurses in the neurosurgery ward whose tremendous kindness, sympathy, and professional competence carried me through those first few frightful days.

. . . My sense of doctoring, I found, had been significantly changed by all that had happened. From medical school on I believed that medicine was something finite and specific, a marathon multiple-choice test in which, as a physician, I was struggling to discover the correct diagnosis and match it to the right treatment. The greater the degree of accuracy I could bring to bear on my continuous skirmishes with the disease, the better the physician I would be. That had certainly been the orientation of my medical training and residency. While I still appreciate accuracy and precision, my illness forcefully broadened my expectations of doctoring. A good physician is one who saw the patient as a whole person, a complex human being, rather than a series of organ systems in various states of repair. This is not an argument against knowledge or even specialization, but rather a recognition, once and for all, that good physicians are more than just Midas Muffler dealers. Generalist or specialist, family practitioner or plastic surgeon, a good doctor needs to love his patient at least a little bit. He needs some curiosity, a touch of fervor, a belief that most people are good and worth knowing. Of course, no practitioner likes – let alone loves – all his patients, and pure technicians function perfectly well in certain areas of medicine, but good patient care requires a sense of loving. If I had any doubt about that before being sick, I have none now.

Mary O'Flaherty Horn, MD was an internist with amyotrophic lateral sclerosis (ALS). In an article in the *Annals of Internal Medicine* series "On Being a Patient", she described the nerve conduction study that diagnosed her illness. As the physician performing the procedure carried on a conversation with the medical students that did not include her, she was made to feel like an object rather than a person. She was comforted by the empathy of the students in the room, one of whom reached out to help her. Her essay lets us see how even the most confident and competent physician can feel paralyzed by fear when faced with a serious illness and, just as important, her experience demonstrates the imbalance of power between patients and doctors – even when the patient is a doctor!

It was apparent on my first introduction to Dr. L. that he was distant. His "good morning" had an automatic quality about it, and my attempts to make pleasant conversation faltered. . . . Suddenly, I was the vehicle for teaching these students about motor neuron pathology. He addressed all concerns to them. I might not have been present except for the obvious need for my muscles. His enthusiasm about the array of abnormal findings was clear as he lectured the students about the "classic findings of ALS". . . . If I moved or said that the needle that he placed in a muscle was uncomfortable, I was regarded with polite but cool irritation. . . . At one point, as I tried to comply with his requests, my gown rose above my hips. As I reached down to correct the problem, he snapped "Don't move!" One of the students, taking pity on me, offered a blanket which I gratefully accepted. The students seemed uncomfortable but remained quiet . . .

As I dressed, I had two immediate thoughts. The first was to escape now and never return. . . . The second was "Thank God I knew I had ALS before I came here, because this would be the cruelest way to find out."

. . . Had I been my usual self, I would not have tolerated such callousness. But when you are sick, the strength and reserves for fighting such treatment are not there . . .

It is a lesson in healing. Although my physicians may not be able to cure my illness, their encouragement, time, patience, and trust build bridges that enable me to cope one day at a time. . . . Physicians are the vital human link that can give patients the strength they require. As the pace of change in medicine quickens, physicians who teach will bear a special responsibility to provide strong examples of empathy and professionalism to students and residents.

Kay Redfield Jamison, PhD, an author and Professor of Psychiatry at Johns Hopkins School of Medicine, wrote a book about her life with a bipolar disorder. In other excerpts in this book she discussed the stigma associated with mental illness. In the following excerpt she talks about the effect of the illness on her life and career.

I have often asked myself whether, given the choice, I would choose to have a manic-depressive illness. If lithium were not available to me, or didn't work for me, the answer would be a simple no. . . . Strangely enough, I think I would choose to have it. It's complicated. Depression is awful beyond words or sounds or images; I would not go through an extended one again. It bleeds relationships through suspicion, lack of confidence and self-respect, the inability to enjoy life. . . . But I honestly believe that because of it I have felt more things, more deeply.

While she was a medical student, **Alison Clay** was hospitalized for a serious asthma attach. During her ICU admission, she discovered the forced helplessness and dependency that illness brings, and she describes how she sometimes felt like an object under discussion rather than a person when she was not included in her physician's conversations with trainees. Her experience gave her a new understanding of how doctors should relate to and communicate with patients.

Intravenous lines run from my body to the ceiling, electrocardiogram leads and the pulse oximeter to the monitor behind me, the facemask to the large tanks of helium and oxygen across the room. I cannot adjust myself in bed without help. Communication is difficult. I do not want to bother the nurses with trivial matters. I depend on those taking care of me to anticipate my needs. . . . These are the details of my life as a patient, things I have not even considered as a student. I judge my caretakers by how they have justified the trust I have placed in them, how they acknowledge my dependence and vulnerability.

Soon several physicians and students file into my room en masse, gather around my bed and stare down at me. I recoil into the recesses of my bed, feeling like a trapped specimen on display as the team presents my case and the attending physician speaks on the benefits of noninvasive ventilation. Instead of speaking above me, I want the team to speak to me. When the team walks out, I want to hear the conclusions drawn by the attending physician.

. . . I long to talk to my physicians not just about my disease, but about how my illness will affect my life now as a medical student and in the future as a resident. But there is little opportunity to discuss these issues. Attending rounds are not the appropriate venue, and pre-rounds is a time for rapid and efficient data collection, not lengthy conversations. I have rarely gone back to a patient's room after rounds to tell the patient what changes we are making in their treatment or to discuss the patient's concerns and feelings. . . . I hope that my physicians are somehow different, more sensitive, more insightful.

Dr. Maurice Raskin wrote about living with ulcerative colitis. He argues that because medical training rewards stoicism and self-control, doctors learn to be intolerant of patients who are anxious or depressed, or whose life is in disarray. They see these characteristics as a sign of personal weakness in the patient, rather than as a normal response to the psychosocial impact of serious illness.

> This raises an important point about the physician's view of the nature of the sick role. I believe that doctors, by and large, associate illness with weakness. We belie our feelings by preferences for certain modes of patient behavior. The dependent, complaining patient is considered weak, stupid, and generally less worthy than the independent patient. The Puritan ethic clearly prevails among US physicians. Patients earn the respect of their caretakers when they are stoical – the "silent sufferers."
>
> . . . Serious illness is something we all fear, consciously or not, because it represents uncertainty and a loss of control. Those who manage their illness with minimal loss of control are admired. Loss of control is particularly dreaded by physicians who are expected to be in control not only of their own lives but of those of others as well. I don't think one can prescribe proper patient behavior. Your caretaker should be good enough to deal appropriately with a wide variety of patterns.
>
> . . . Finally, how should one try to behave as a patient and, more important, does this tell us something about how we should, perhaps, treat our own patients? . . . In general, I now believe that patients should be encouraged to retain as much control over their care as they want and are capable of handling. There is no place in the practice of medicine for paternalism. . . . We do no public service by encouraging dependency in competent adults.
>
> Has illness changed me as a person? I went through an experience as a young adult that most people do not encounter until they have reached an advanced age. In a sense, then, I have been aged by illness. I have become more appreciative of the world around me and less concerned about what people think about me. I am more self-reliant.
>
> I feel closer to the relatives and friends who have shared my plight. And I hope I have become just a bit wiser. After all, it would have been a shame to have been at the gates of hell and not learned from the journey.

Dr. David Hein wrote about his experience with Crohn's disease:

I truly believe that having lived these past 50 years in the shadow of personal health problems, becoming aware of my reactions to them, and working through difficult solutions have been a greater advantage than disadvantage to me as a physician and as a human being.

Dr. Harvey Mandell edited a book of essays, *When Doctors Get Sick*, written by physicians about their experience with illness. In the following excerpt, he discusses how his life was changed by the diagnosis of malignant melanoma:

At first my illness and surgery gave me more patience with patients who were frightened or couldn't wait a reasonable time for laboratory and imaging tests to come back, but eventually that wore off and I guess in the long run I was not more affable than before. For a while it made me better with people who acted in unpleasant ways or who seemed hostile at first meeting. It gave me pause to wonder if their behaviors were governed at least in part by something they weren't sharing with me. I did develop permanently more feeling and understanding for those who failed to get the same sort of support from their spouses that I did.

Charles Kleinman, MD, a pediatric cardiologist at a prestigious and high-pressured academic medical school, was diagnosed with Hodgkin's disease early in his career. His experience led him to a new understanding of the important role of doctors as patient advocates, which he describes eloquently as follows:

At the same time, I have been changed as a physician. I have always thought that I have a large measure of compassion and empathy, but I have found that it is much easier to walk alongside a gurney than to lie on one.

I have learned how easy it is to become a nameless, seemingly ignored entity, with explanation rarely offered unless demanded. I know of the need for each patient to have an advocate. In this regard, I have redoubled my efforts to communicate fully with patients and their parents. The patient in the hospital and his family often live from one visit to the next of their physician. There is no reason why there should not be communication daily, and more often if necessary.

Most families come to the hospital seeking efficient, professional care. They want to be cared for by people who are gentle, compassionate, and competent. They are not usually looking for a buddy who introduces him- or herself by first name, the way your waiter for the evening does so at the local Steak and Brew.

I have also learned that while patients and their families want to think their doctor is all-knowing and all-seeing, they also want him to be honest.

. . . During the months following the diagnosis of Hodgkin's disease, I wore the diagnosis on my sleeve. I felt that it was good for me and good for the children in the oncology clinic to speak to newly diagnosed patients with Hodgkin's so I could tell them what to expect. . . . It soon became clear to me that I was not ready to take on such a burden as a regular habit. I, frankly, do not know enough about the disease to really counsel someone, and am still vulnerable enough to imagine developing some of the complications that less fortunate patients develop.

. . . Even if all goes well, as appears likely, I will never be happy that my family and I have gone through the travails of the past five years. Nonetheless, much good has come from this experience. I would like to think that eventually I would have reordered my priorities, placing family and humanism above some of the more tangible, yet less meaningful goals that one may have in life.

Despite the diagnosis of end-stage renal disease as a young man, **Dr. Peter Lunden** finished college and medical school while on dialysis, and then went on to subspecialize in nephrology. In the following passage, he explains how his life on dialysis allowed him to identify with the life of his patients with end-stage renal disease. This shared experience gave him insights into the behavior of his patients who were sometimes discouraged, unengaged, noncompliant, or without hope. He understood the complicated interpersonal dynamics between the healthcare providers, who control dialysis scheduling and treatment, and the patients, who can feel powerless and vulnerable. He wrote the following essay when he was 42 years of age

I am a nephrologist who is also a 20-year veteran of hemodialysis. I was a patient before I was a doctor. I am comfortable with both roles, and each has taught me ways to augment the other. Having a chronic illness has offered me a number of advantages in my medical practice. It has helped me understand the thinking processes and motivations, fears and concerns of being a patient. I have learned to combine the patient's insights with the knowledge and technical skills of a physician. Being a patient has taught me to modify my approach to diagnosis and treatment of diseases in ways that stress prevention and minimize harm. Most important for people with a health problem is regaining some predictability in living.

While the healthy person tends to suffer through minor ailments with a minimum of fuss, the chronically ill have a tendency to give significance to almost every new bodily discomfort and pay them more attention than they deserve. . . . It is important to assure patients of your alertness and concern. Caring for the chronically ill is often a difficult and trying task, and thus unpleasant to many doctors. Dealing with these patients requires patience and sustained concern.

What I have gained from being a patient is the ability to feel extremely comfortable with patients, particularly those with a similar problem. We share an experience. They feel confident that when I say that I know what they are going through, they know it to be true. I am most relaxed when speaking at their meetings about commonly shared problems. I am not put off when they are angry or depressed about what has happened to them. They are facing one of life's major traumas and are entitled to react accordingly. I have learned patience and understanding, and have found myself willing to go the extra distance with the angry or noncompliant patient.

. . . Like the dying individuals that they are, patients with renal failure need to go through several stages of adaptation before they come to an acceptance of their fate. . . . The early stages of anger come as the individual struggles to get back in control. Many dialysis patients find themselves in the position where control is almost entirely in the hands of doctors and nurses, and the only choices for independence are self-dialysis or kidney transplant.

Dr. Ronald Karpick is a pulmonologist who was treated for tuberculosis:

I try not to hospitalize patients, not because of DRGs but because of the hospital's impact on their lives. I can appreciate the loss of control, the dehumanization, the cost. I don't usually discuss my personal history with patients, but if they appear to be having a particularly hard time adjusting, I will tell them . . .

Living and working with significant depression helped **Dr. Louise Redmond** to understand and meet the needs of her own patients. It increased her sensitivity to the diagnosis of depression in her own practice, and the empathy she felt for the vulnerability caused by her patients' illness:

> I often wonder if my illness has helped or harmed me in my dealing with patients. I believe depressed people find each other and often seek help from people who have been depressed themselves. . . . I believe that experiencing illness has heightened my sensitivity to many other problems. It is very difficult to project an impersonal image when one is so acutely aware of one's own vulnerability. My dealing with patients must be more personal; I simply cannot take myself too seriously. And understanding my own illness and my reluctance to use or trust health care provides me, I believe, with an advantage over my less vulnerable colleagues. The human condition afflicts us all in one way or another. If I have this weakness, I also have some talent, and I will use it to help my patients as my therapist helped me. . . . To listen, to empathize, to walk in my patient's shoes, weak though I may be – these are the measures of my worth as a physician healer.

Dr. Rosemary MacKenzie also lived with a significant depression at a time when it was associated with so much stigma that physicians rarely sought treatment. She speaks about how her illness changed her perspective on her own life:

> My illness gave me a sense of perspective during which I sorted out my priorities. It also gave me a sense of mortality and time passing, which has given me the impetus to do things which I had formerly only thought about. . . . It is difficult to think about these four years as anything more than a waste of my life. . . . In retrospect, I became quite frightened. I lost four years because I would not or could not ask for help. I think that I was at considerable risk of dying; I am quite appalled when I think of that. I hope I wouldn't ever do that again. . . . I hope that by talking about it and writing about it, I may make somebody, somewhere talk about it rather than pick up a bottle of pills. . . . It would be a terrible thing to die of pride.

Dr. Lawrence Freedman, an internist and professor of medicine, was hospitalized for a traumatic brain injury that caused significant memory loss and impaired his cognitive function. His recovery was slow, his physicians could not tell him whether he would return to full function, and the uncertainty left him feeling anxious and isolated. His disability had profound effects on his ability to function at home and at work, and on his self-image. Physicians who were technically excellent didn't offer him the information he needed to live with his disability, and psychosocial support was offered haphazardly or not at all. In the following excerpt, he discusses the patient's need for information, support, and encouragement, and the importance of including this training in medical education:

I realized that my physicians had not addressed the psychological conse-quences of my injury, nor had they prepared or advised my family about the inevitable anxiety that would accompany recovery. I felt intensely alone with my worries, too frightened, protective, and too insecure to do anything but worry more. . . . In retrospect, I realized that the more I recovered, the more frightening and shaking the whole event seemed and the more I worried.

. . . What did I miss most as a patient recovering from a cerebral con-cussion? I wanted my physician to talk to me; I needed them to talk to me, particularly as I improved and knew what I wanted to discuss. . . . As I look back, I know that I was unaware of this need at the time, and was therefore incapable of expressing it. . . . I would have wanted to hear about the experiences to be anticipated after such an injury, about their evolution, about their impact on me personally and professionally. I would have benefited from the identification of any signs of progress and improvement, and encouragement as to the probability of full recovery.

. . . I would have benefited from the opportunity to express concerns and ask questions. It is clear to me, however, that I would not have gotten to personal issues without having first developed a relationship of trust with my physicians, and such relationships take time to develop.

I realize, as I write, that I sound like the army of patients who have expressed and continue to express these sentiments. But why is this dimension of care so lacking? Several reasons come to mind. Perhaps one apparent reason is that physicians are poorly compensated for their time unless they carry out well-codified, remunerative procedures.

Another reason is that the human aspects of illness and medical care are not infused with the attention and emphasis that they deserve. In the physician, human understanding and involvement is presumed to be inborn and then enhanced by the experience – and sometimes it is. But "sometimes" is not enough, and most important, is not predictable. The reality is that such care requires instruction and guidance – elements that are conspicuously absent from our traditional formal medical teaching.

. . . Somehow, coincident with the spectacular advances in science and medicine in recent years, the physicians is perceived as being less aware of/ competent to manage the human aspects of medical care.

. . . I remember when, during the recovery from my concussion, I realized that I no longer understood or felt music. It was then that I knew that something was wrong with me. As I reflect upon the emphasis in medicine today and the forces pushing it in the direction in which it is evolving, I no longer understand the music; I know something is wrong.

Conclusions

After years of practice, when I get home in the evening I still look forward to scanning the titles in the medical journals that arrive each day, searching for articles that give me new insights into the mechanisms of diseases I have treated for years, offer new treatment options, or shake up assumptions about what I thought I knew about medicine. But now, as I page through the *New England Journal of Medicine*, *JAMA*, or the *Annals of Internal Medicine*, I find that the articles I read first are the essays of physicians and patients about the day-to-day practice of medicine. When I am tired and feeling a little drained, these are the articles that make me laugh, smile, relax, and reflect about the significant but sometimes unnoticed things that happen each day as I care for patients.

These interactions with patients offer us insights into who we are as people, what leads to happiness, and how tenuous our hold on security and happiness is. Years of conversations with patients about their illnesses and their lives show us that vulnerability, whether it is due to illness, financial stresses, or personal loss, is not the exception but the rule. Very few professions, other than medicine, allow such an unguarded view into the most private parts of people's lives and thoughts, and few offer as much opportunity to learn and to help. It is a tremendous privilege and responsibility.

But, over time, we often fail to recognize the importance of what is happening in front of us, every day. At some point during our professional careers, as we become busier, more tired, and more distracted, the profound can seem routine. When we rush past the most vulnerable moments in people's lives without recognizing them, when we treat patients and colleagues brusquely, or stop noticing the impact of our actions, we lose a little of our humanity. And this loss impacts not only on our interactions with patients, but also on our personal relationships and, eventually, our self-esteem.

Atul Gawande and Rita Charon, two physicians who write about the practice of medicine, advise medical students to write about their experiences in medicine. Writing, whether it is to prepare a presentation or to collect your thoughts about interactions with patients, focuses your thinking and allows you to see what you might not notice otherwise. Time for reflection is difficult to find in medical training or practice, but observations about human nature, our reactions to the people we meet, and the humor and humanity in these interactions make the day-to-day practice of medicine more enjoyable and put the frustrations into perspective. The thoughtful essays of patients and practitioners remind us of the unique rewards of medicine and the potentially profound impact of our actions on the lives of the people we care for in the same way that articles about new scientific advances tweak our intellectual curiosity and motivate us to provide the best medical treatment.

So, the challenge as you start practice is to make sure that there is enough quiet time in your professional career for you to have a chance to notice, listen, wonder, and maybe even write about the important things that happen every week. This peaceful time to clear your mind and reflect about people, society, values, and your own actions and reactions will help you to keep the important things in perspective, and will allow you to be the physician you hope to be, as Dr. Hines describes in the excerpt that follows.

> Not until much after he died, as I was preparing a talk for premed students, did I come to realize that Guillermo [a patient with HIV] was as beneficial to my mental health as I was to his. For instance, yesterday in the office an off-duty police officer handed me a summons to appear in court for a case I couldn't even recall. In the mail, I found notices from my insurance carrier that my premiums were doubling, a silly graph showing my length of stay at the hospital compared to other doctors, and an article detailing the Medicare cuts that Congress has in store for next year. Beautiful! Was it just me or is the world about to implode? It was enough to make me suicidal. That is when Guillermo comes to my rescue.
>
> When the "mierda de perro" (his expression for BS) gets too thick, I look for something to remind me why I went into this profession in the first

place. Guillermo showed me what impact a simple gesture could have on another individual. Patients helping doctors with their problems? Now that was a different way of looking at it. Guillermo showed me that in giving, you also receive. Suddenly, the sorry state of medical affairs was relegated to the back seat on the bus that is my brain – far behind family, friends, did I feed the fish that morning, and the new dent my daughter added to my left front bumper. I think we all have our Guillermos, and we should honor them whenever the "mierda" gets too deep.

David W. Hines, MD

References and Additional Reading

*Denotes a memoir or essay.

Association of American Medical Colleges. *Learning Objectives for Medical Student Education: Guidelines for Medical Schools.* Washington, DC: AAMC; 1998.

Barr D. A time to listen. *Ann Intern Med.* 2004; **140:** 144.

Bergsma J. *Doctors and Patients: strategies in long-term illness.* Dordrecht, The Netherlands: Kluwer Academic Publishers; 1997.

*Brice JA. Ulcerative colitis and avascular necrosis of the hips. In: Mandell H, Spiro H, editors. *When Doctors Get Sick.* New York: Plenum Medical Book Company; 1987.

Cassel E. The nature of suffering and the goals of medicine. *NEJM.* 1982; **306:** 639–45.

Cassel E. *The Nature of Suffering and the Goals of Medicine.* New York: Oxford University Press; 1991.

Cassel J. *The Healer's Art: a new approach to the doctor–patient relationship.* New York: JB Lippincott; 1976.

Charmaz K. *Good Days, Bad Days: the self in chronic illness and time.* New Brunswick, NJ: Rutgers University Press; 1991.

Chen D. It's only 50 cents. *Ann Intern Med.* 2001; **135:** 1087–8.

*Chorost M. *Rebuilt: my journey back to the hearing world.* New York: Houghton Mifflin Co.; 2005.

*Clay A. The medical student as patient. *Ann Intern Med.* 1999; **131:** 225–6.

Coles R, editor. *William Carlos Williams: the doctor stories.* New York: New Directions Books; 1984.

Coles R, Testa R, editors. *A Life in Medicine: a literary anthology.* New York: The New York Press; 2002.

Cousins N. Physician as humanist. In: Reiser D, Rosen D, editors. *Medicine as a Human Experience.* Rockville, MD: Aspen Publishers; 1984.

Das Gupta S, Charon R. Personal illness narratives: using reflective writing to teach empathy. *Acad Med.* 2004; **79:** 351–6.

*Frank A. *At the Will of the Body: reflections on illness*. New York: Houghton Mifflin Company; 1991.

Frankel D, Liebman CJ. Words that heal. *Ann Intern Med.* 2004; **140:** 482.

*Freedman L. Traumatic brain injury. In: Mandell H, Spiro H, editors. *When Doctors Get Sick*. New York: Plenum Medical Book Company; 1987.

Gawande A. *Complications: a surgeon's notes on an imperfect science*. New York: Henry Holt and Co.; 2002.

Gawande A. *Better: a surgeon's notes on performance*. New York: Henry Holt and Co.; 2007.

Gilbert D. *Stumbling on Happiness*. New York: Alfred A. Knopf; 2006.

Goodman J. Nobility. *Ann Intern Med.* 2001; **134:** 621–2.

Groopman J. *How People Prevail in the Face of Illness: the anatomy of hope*. New York: Random House; 2004.

*Hein D. Crohn's disease. In: Mandell H, Spiro H, editors. *When Doctors Get Sick*. New York: Plenum Medical Book Company; 1987.

Herscheimer A. Helping patients take responsibility for their own health. *Ann Intern Med.* 2001; **135:** 51–2.

Hines D. Maestro Guillermo. *Ann Intern Med.* 2007; **147:** 670.

Horowitz CR, Suchman AL, Branch WT *et al.* What do doctors find meaningful about their work? *Ann Intern Med.* 2003; **138:** 772–5.

*Karpick R. Tuberculosis. In: Mandell H, Spiro H, editors. *When Doctors Get Sick*. New York: Plenum Medical Book Company; 1987.

Kenyon J. *Otherwise: new and selected poems*. St Paul, MN: Graywolf Press; 1996.

Kleinman A. *The Illness Narratives: suffering, healing, and the human condition*. New York: Basic Books; 1988.

*Kleinman C. Hodgkin's disease. In: Mandell H, Spiro H, editors. *When Doctors Get Sick*. New York: Plenum Medical Book Company; 1987.

*Kooser T. *Local Wonders: seasons in the Bohemian Alps*. Lincoln, NE: University of Nebraska Press; 2002.

Levasseur J, Vance D. Doctors, patients and empathy. In: Spiro H, Peschel E, McCrea Curnen MG *et al.*, editors. *Empathy and the Practice of Medicine*. New Haven, CT: Yale University Press; 1993.

*Lunden P. Chronic renal failure and hemodialysis. In: Mandell H, Spiro H, editors. *When Doctors Get Sick*. New York: Plenum Medical Book Company; 1987.

*Lynn J. Travels in the Valley of the Shadow. In: Spiro H, Peschel E, McCrea Curnen MG *et al.*, editors. *Empathy and the Practice of Medicine*. New Haven, CT: Yale University Press; 1993.

*MacKenzie A. Depression. In: Mandell H, Spiro H, editors. *When Doctors Get Sick*. New York: Plenum Medical Book Company; 1987.

*Mandell H. Maliganant melanoma. In: Mandell H, Spiro H, editors. *When Doctors Get Sick*. New York: Plenum Medical Book Company; 1987.

*Mandell H, Spiro H, editors. *When Doctors Get Sick*. New York: Plenum Medical Book Company; 1987.

Morowitz HJ. The pre-med as a metaphor of antipathy. In: Spiro H, Peschel E, McCrea Curnen MG *et al.*, editors. *Empathy and the Practice of Medicine*. New Haven, CT: Yale University Press; 1993.

*Mullan F. *Vital Signs, A Young Doctor's Struggle with Cancer*. New York: Dell Publishing Co.; 1975.

Newton BW, Barber LB, Clardy J, Cleveland E, O'Sullivan P. Is there a hardening of the heart during medical school? *Acad Med*. 2008; **83**: 224–49.

*Nixon N, Nixon B, editors. *People with AIDS*. Boston, MA: David Godine Publishers, Inc.; 1991.

*O'Flaherty Horn M. The other side of the bedrail. *Ann Intern Med*. 1999; **130**: 940–1.

Power P, Dell Orto A. *Families Living with Chronic Illness and Disability: interventions, challenges, and opportunities*. New York: Springer Publishing Co.; 2004.

*Price R. *A Whole New Life: an illness and a healing*. New York: Atheneum; 1982.

*Rabin D, Rabin P, Rabin R. Compounding the ordeal of ALS: isolation from my fellow physicians. *NEJM*. 1962; **307**: 506–9.

Raj YP. Lessons from a label maker. *Ann Intern Med*. 2005; **143**: 686–7.

*Raskin M. Ulcerative colitis. In: Mandell H, Spiro H, editors. *When Doctors Get Sick*. New York: Plenum Medical Book Company; 1987.

*Redfield Jamison K. *An Unquiet Mind: a memoir of moods and madness*. New York: Alfred A. Knopf; 1995.

*Redmond L. Depression. In: Mandell H, Spiro H, editors. *When Doctors Get Sick*. New York: Plenum Medical Book Company; 1987.

*Reiser D, Rosen D. *Medicine as a Human Experience*. Rockville, MD: Aspen Publishers; 1984.

Reynolds R, Stone J, editors. *On Doctoring: stories, poems, and essays*. New York: Simon and Schuster; 2001.

Royer A. *Living with Chronic Illness: social and psychological dimensions*. Westport, CT: Praeger Publishers; 1998.

*Rucker A. *The Best Seat in the House: how I woke up one Tuesday and was paralyzed for life*. New York: HarperCollins Publishers; 2007.

*Scott L. Ulcerative colitis. In: Mandell H, Spiro H, editors. *When Doctors Get Sick*. New York: Plenum Medical Book Company; 1987.

Sontag S. *Illness as a Metaphor*. New York: Farrar, Strauss, and Giroux; 1978.

Spiro H, Peschel E, McCrea Curnen GM *et al.*, editors. *Empathy and the Practice of Medicine*. New Haven, CT: Yale University Press; 1993.

*Stein M. *The Lonely Patient: how we experience illness.* New York: HarperCollins Publishers; 2007.

*Styron W. *Darkness Visible: a memoir of madness.* New York: Random House; 1990.

Thomas L. *The Youngest Science: Notes of a Medicine-Watcher.* New York: Viking Press; 1983.

Tumulty P. The art of healing. *Johns Hopkins Med J.* 1978; **143:** 140–3.

*Updike J. *Self-Consciousness: memoirs.* New York: Alfred A. Knopf; 1989.

Verghese A. The physician as storyteller. *Ann Intern Med.* 2001; **135:** 1012–17.

Verghese A. Empathy and the literary imagination. *Ann Intern Med.* 2002; **137:** 627–9.

Watts D. *Bedside Manners.* New York: Harmony Books; 2005.

Welsh L, Betancourt M. *Chronic Illness and the Family: a guide for living every day.* Holbrook, MA: Adams Media Corp.; 1996.

Wheby MS. An examination of conscience. *Ann Intern Med.* 2002; **136:** 486–7.

William WC. *The Autobiography of William Carlos Williams.* New York: New Directions Books; 1967.

*Wolfson P. *Moonrise: one family, genetic identity, and muscular dystrophy.* New York: St Martin's Press; 2003.

*Young Bradshaw D. A visit to the doctor. *Ann Intern Med.* 1999; **131:** 627–8.

*Zola IK. *Missing Pieces: a chronicle of living with disability.* Philadelphia, PA: Temple University Press; 1982.

Additional Resources

There are other excellent resources about the psychosocial impact of illness, how to interview and communicate with patients, how to talk to patients about disability and end-of-life care, and professionalism. Some are them are listed here.

Burgsma J. _Doctors and Patients: strategies in long-term illness._ Dordrecht, The Netherlands: Kluwer Academic Publishers; 1997.

Cassell EJ. _Talking with Patients: the theory of doctor–patient communication._ Boston, MA: MIT Press; 1985.

Desmond J, Copeland LR. _Communicating with Today's Patient: essentials to save time, decrease risk, and increase patient compliance._ San Francisco, CA: Jossey-Bass Publishers; 2000.

Hahn RA. _Sickness and Healing: an anthropological perspective._ New Haven, CT: Yale University Press; 1995.

Platt FW, Gordon GH. _Field Guide to the Difficult Patient Interview._ New York: Lippincott Williams and Wilkens; 1999.

Roter DL, Hall JA. _Doctors Talking with Patients, Patients Talking with Doctors: improving communication in medical visits._ Westport, CT: Auburn House; 1993.

Silverman J, Kurtz S, Draper J. _Skills for Communicating with Patients._ Oxford: Radcliffe Medical Press; 1999.

Course Description

Course Overview

This book was developed for a four-week seminar for senior medical students but can also be adapted for classes in medical humanities and doctor–patient communication. The course is broken up into two sections. The first discusses the experience of serious illness from the patient's point of view, and emphasizes the distinction between understanding disease and understanding the personal impact of illness. Using the patient's own words, the readings and interviews illustrate how a person's life is profoundly changed by serious illness. They describe the long-term impact of fear, vulnerability, uncertainty, and loss of control on self-image, roles, relationships, and psychological well-being.

The second part of the course reviews the physician's role in educating, advising, and counseling patients about medical and psychosocial issues. Techniques for discussing difficult psychosocial issues are reviewed, and the role of physician as a patient advocate is emphasized.

Suggested readings include three memoirs about illness (one a week) over the first three weeks of the seminar and the relevant parts of this book. The memoirs are listed in *References and Additional Reading* and are designated by an asterisk. Additional readings are listed for some sections.

Two written assignments are suggested. The first is a "Thought Experiment" – an essay in which the writer will discuss how a serious illness would impact their life, relationships, and professional and personal goals. The second is a final paper in which the writer will synthesize the themes discussed in the class with insights from the patient interviews and readings. Outlines for both writing assignments are provided in later chapters.

Topics for class discussions are listed in the next section. In each section, a new theme is introduced. The discussion springs from the memoirs, the additional reading assignments, the patient interviews, and, perhaps most important for those students who have had some clinical experience, the interactions observed between patients and doctors in the hospital and clinics. Suggestions for questions to facilitate the discussions are also given under each topic.

For the first few weeks, about every other class begins with a patient interview. First-hand accounts of illness often convey the emotional impact of illness in a way that written material cannot. Two group patient interviews are recommended in the first few weeks of the class. Once everyone is comfortable with the interview and questions, one or two one-on-one patient interviews should be completed in the last weeks of the course.

Patients who are invited to the group interviews should understand that they will be asked about the personal aspects of living with illness. After introductions, the facilitator will start the interview by asking the patient to tell the group how the illness began and how it was diagnosed. Then the discussion can be opened up to include the psychosocial issues with participation from the whole group. Suggested questions for the interviews are provided in a later chapter.

These sessions usually last about 90 minutes, with half the time spent with the patient and the remaining time for discussion. Starting the discussion right after the interview captures ideas and impressions while they are still fresh. For each interview, one student will be asked to be the host and to facilitate the interview, and another student will lead the class discussion. Suggestions for questions for the interviews and for discussion are listed under that session, but each interview will bring up unique and unexpected issues.

Depending on the time available for the course, two optional sessions are offered – one on patient decision making and the other on medical error.

Themes and Readings

SESSION 1

1 Course overview: In the first session, start by reviewing the goals of the class and the expectations for readings, interview, and writing assignments.

2 Review reading assignments for next session:

   Book Section 1: *The Impact of Illness on Identity, Self-Esteem, Roles, and Relationships.*

   First memoir (suggested books for the first 3 weeks include the memoirs of Fitzhugh Mullan, Reynolds Price, Kay Redfield Jamison, and Arthur Frank).

   Review the questions in the *Guide to Readings.*

3 Review writing assignments:

   Discussion of the essay *My Life with Serious Illness* to be completed by Session 6.

   Final paper to be completed by Session 8.

SESSION 2

1 Start with group patient interview.

2 Discussion of the first topic: The impact of serious illness on the person: identity, self-esteem, roles, and relationships.

The first chapter opens with this quote from Arthur Frank:

> *Critical illness leaves no aspect of life unchanged. . . . Your relationships, your work, your sense of who you are and who you might become, your sense of what life is and what it ought to be – these all change and the change is terrifying. Twice, as I realized how ill I was, I saw these changes coming and was overwhelmed by them.*

How does this statement apply to the author of the memoir you are reading? How was the author's life changed by illness?

Later in the chapter, there is another quote from Dr. Frank:

> *Illness excuses people from their normal responsibilities, but the cost of being excused is greater than it appears at first. An excuse is also an exclusion.*

What does he mean by exclusion? How do the other readings demonstrate this idea?

What is Arthur Frank suggesting when he says *"Illness can crowd out talk"?*

3   Group discussion of the patient interview.

How did the patient view their doctor? Other doctors? The medical care delivery system (hospitals, clinics, ancillaries, testing, technology)?

Compare and contrast the patient's experience and those described in the class readings and memoirs.

What explains these differences (the type of illness, the patient's personality, medical or life experience, other)?

Do you think the patient was completely honest in all their answers? What might have limited what they were willing or able to say?

SESSION 3

1   Reading assignments to be completed by this class:

   ℘ Second memoir.

   ℘ Book Section 1: *Emotional Responses to Serious Illness.*

   ℘ Additional readings.

- *The Other Side of the Bedrail*, by Mary O'Flaherty-Horn
- *Medical Student as Patient*, by Alison Clay
- *It's Only 50 Cents*, by Daniel Chen

2 Topics for discussion.

- Discuss the themes of psychological impact of illness as demonstrated in the patient interview, memoirs, and articles.

- How does the following comment by Drs. Reiser and Rosen apply to the responses to illness described in the memoirs you have read?
  - *How the individual handles being sick reflects his attitudes, defenses, strengths, weaknesses, and philosophy of life.*

- What is Dr. O'Flaherty-Horn describing in this excerpt?
  - *I had certainly been in large medical centers before; therefore, there was no reason to feel overwhelmed. I myself am a well-trained internist from a large university – I knew the scene – but this summer morning was different. I was tired and scared. Just two weeks before I had been told that the slurred speech that had been progressing for several months was probably caused by amyotrophic lateral sclerosis (ALS). They'd said 2 to 5 years and, as a physician, I knew all too well the grim prognosis and disheartening lack of therapy associated with my diagnosis.*

- Why was the daily newspaper so important to the patient in the essay, *It's Only 50 Cents*?

- How does the impact of fear, anxiety, vulnerability, and loss of control change patients' behavior at home or in the hospital or doctor's office? Give some examples.

SESSION 4

1 Second group interview.

2 Discussion of readings and interviews.

- What was the personal impact of the illness on the patient who was interviewed?

    ⚘ What was the most memorable or surprising part of the interview?

    ⚘ Was the patient changed by their illness? Why or why not?

    ⚘ Compare and contrast the personal impact of illness on this patient and other patients interviewed and/or the authors of the articles and memoirs.

    ⚘ Did the patient talk about the imbalance in power between doctors and patients? How did it affect their behavior and the doctor–patient relationship?

SESSION 5

1   Readings to be completed by these classes.

    ⚘ Third memoir.

    ⚘ Book Section 1: *Coping and Renewal* and *Aftermath: Life after Illness*.

2   Topics for discussion.

    ⚘ Discuss the lasting effects of illness on the people interviewed and the authors.
       ⌣ What aspects of the patient's personality, environment, or supports helped them to deal with the changes brought on by illness?
       ⌣ What aspects of illness lead to anxiety, depression, anger, guilt, or burnout? In what ways do patients demonstrate these emotions in the medical setting?

SESSION 6

⚘ Discuss the *Thought Experiment*. How would illness affect your life? Compare your reactions with those of the authors of the memoirs and the patients interviewed.

⚘ Discuss the individual patient interviews and final paper to be done in the following week(s).

SESSION 7

1   Readings:

- ✐ Sections 2 and 3: *The Doctor's Role* and *Reflections of Doctors on Illness, Medical Training, and Clinical Care*.

- ✐ Additional readings.
  - ⌐ *Can You Teach Compassion?* By Jerome Lowenstein (from Coles R, Testa R, editors. *A Life in Medicine: a Literary Anthology*).
  - ⌐ *Compounding the Ordeal of ALS: Isolation from my Fellow Physicians*, by David Rabin.
  - ⌐ *A Time to Listen*, by Donald Barr.
  - ⌐ *Step by Step*, by Jerome Groopman (from *The Anatomy of Hope: How People Prevail in the Face of Illness*).
  - ⌐ *A Visit to the Doctor*, by Deborah Young Bradshaw.
  - ⌐ *An Examination of Conscience*, by Munsey Wheby.
  - ⌐ *Lessons from a Label Maker*, by Gary Hoffman and Carol Lightfoot.
  - ⌐ *The Other Side of the Bedrail*, by Mary O'Flaherty-Horn.

2   Group discussion:

- ✐ Education.
  - ⌐ What information would you want from your physician if you discovered that you had a serious illness?
  - ⌐ Why was the patient in the article *Lessons from a Label Maker* noncompliant with medication?
  - ⌐ In the essay entitled *The Bell Curve*, a physician who treats patients with cystic fibrosis says "The thing about patients with CF is that they are good scientists. They always experiment. We have to help them interpret what they experience as they experiment." What is he talking about? How did the doctor–patient relationship and patient education affect the outcomes of patients at different centers treating cystic fibrosis?
  - ⌐ How much time have you spent educating patients about their illness during your clinical rotations? What were the barriers to these discussions?

- ✐ Communication.
  - ⌐ What are the barriers to effective communication between doctors and patients?

- What was the problem with communication in the essays *Lessons from a Label Maker, A Visit to the Doctor, Compounding the Ordeal of ALS: Isolation from My Fellow Physicians, A Time to Listen, The Other Side of the Bedrail,* and *Step by Step*? What did the physicians learn about talking to patients?
- Discuss clinical situations where you felt embarrassed by the interaction between the doctors and the patients, or by the way that a patient was being treated. Do you have any thoughts about why the interaction went so badly?
- Discuss clinical situations where you saw very positive interactions between doctors and patients. Why do you think the interaction went so well?
- Discuss clinical interactions where you were unsure of what to say to a patient in distress.

- Counseling.
  - Discuss the suggestions for talking with patients about psychosocial issues outlined in the book. What were the strengths and limitations? What have you observed that is helpful?
  - What would you expect and find helpful if you were ill?
  - Discuss your reactions to the last section of the book, on physicians' reflections on illness. What did they learn that they didn't learn during their medical training? Why didn't they learn it during their training?

SESSION 8

1 Discuss individual patient interviews.
- What did you learn?
- What was helpful?
- What did not go well and why?

2 Overview of the course.
- What did they find most and least helpful in the course?
- Has anything changed in the way they think they would interact with patients with serious illness?
- What are the unresolved issues, critiques of the course or course materials?

⬧ End the course with a reading of the excerpt from the last physician reflection by Dr. Lawrence Friedman.

OPTIONAL TOPICS
SESSION 9: PATIENT DECISION MAKING

⬧ Reading:
  — *Whose Body Is It Anyway?* by Atul Gawande (from *Complications*).
  — *Helping Patients Take Responsibility for Their Own Health*, by Andrew Herscheimer.

⬧ Topics for discussion.
  — Why is it important for patients to take an active role in medical decision making?
  — What tools do patients need to take an active role?
  — What do doctors and allied health providers do that encourages or discourages patient participation?
  — How do you respond to patients who will not take an active role?

SESSION 10: MISTAKES

⬧ Readings:
  — *Flu Shot*, by David Watts.
  — *Mistakes*, by David Hilfiker (from *On Doctoring: Stories, Poems, and Essays*).
  — *When Good Doctors Go Bad*, by Atul Gawande (from *Complications*).
  — *The Case of the Red Leg*, by Atul Gawande (from *Complications*).
  — *Nobility*, by James Goodman.
  — *Words that Heal*, by Douglas Frankel, JD, and Carol J. Liebman, JD.

⬧ Topics for discussion.
  — Medical errors are inevitable. What is their impact on patients and physicians?
  — How do you think you will deal with errors you make in patient care (both errors of commission and those of omission)?
  — How would you discuss expected complications with patients and their families?

Guide to Readings

Choose three books from the references that are personal narratives about illness. For each book, think about each of the following questions:

1   Describe the author's reaction to the diagnosis of their illness. If you were diagnosed with that illness, do you think that your response would have been different?

2   Describe how the illness affected:
    a) the author's self-image and self worth
    b) their personal relationships
    c) their roles at home
    d) their roles at work
    e) their outlook on life.

3   Did the author discuss fear, anxiety, anger, guilt, depression, or burnout?

4   What were the most difficult challenges for the author in living with their illness?

5   What aspects of their life, personality, or relationships were most helpful in dealing with their illness?

6   Were they active or passive participants in their care?

7   Do you think that they were changed by their illness? If so, how?

8   Were there any positive aspects to living with the illness?

9   What was your impression of their physicians and medical care?

10   What annoyed you about the author?

11   What did you admire about the author?

12 Did you think that there was anything that they could or should have done differently in living with their illness? What would you have done differently?

13 Compare and contrast the authors of the three books you read in three of the areas listed above.

14 Which book did you find most helpful in improving your understanding of the personal impact of illness? Why?

Guide to Patient Interviews

As part of this course, you will talk to patients about the impact of illness on their life. This is your opportunity to take a little more time to delve into the social history than you had (or will have) during your clinical rotations. The first interviews will be in groups, and then you will conduct one or two individual interviews.

FINDING A PATIENT TO INTERVIEW

Look for a patient who is medically stable, able to give a good history, and who has lived with a serious illness for a while. What is the definition of serious illness? Try to find someone whose illness was life-threatening, disabling, or life-changing – altering the course of their life and/or causing periods of hospitalization or disability.

When you ask a patient whether you can talk with them, identify yourself as a student or trainee and let them know that you are learning about the personal impact of illness on people and their families. They should understand that you will be asking them personal questions about their self-image, relationships, and work.

SETTING FOR THE INTERVIEW

Find a quiet room (if possible), and sit at eye level with the person you are interviewing. Make sure that both you and the patient are comfortable.

THINGS TO CONSIDER AS YOU CONDUCT THE INTERVIEW

- You will be talking to people from diverse backgrounds, with different illnesses, educational backgrounds, and personal and family supports. They will be at various stages in their adjustment to their illness.

- Try to interview the patient alone, without family members present initially, because they may be less likely to talk about emotional issues or struggles in front of relatives.

- Remember to dress appropriately as a sign of respect.

- Don't try to discuss all of the issues listed with every patient. Some people will be much more responsive to some questions, so spend more time on those. Generally, the interviews should last about 45 minutes.

- Patients generally feel very comfortable talking to medical students and trainees. They see you as open and well intentioned, and they want to help you so that you will take better care of people like them who are ill. They probably think of you as more sympathetic and less threatening than most other medical professionals with whom they have contact. You may be surprised at their willingness to tell you about very personal aspects of their life.

- Many people who have been seriously ill felt very lonely during their illness and want to tell their story so that doctors will address these psychosocial issues with other patients. It gives the illness meaning, and there is great consolation in knowing that their experience may help someone else. They may never have discussed these psychosocial issues with anyone before – not even with their family, friends, or physicians. This could be the first time anyone has asked them. You may discover that you have opened Pandora's Box and the patient will talk at length – perhaps more than you can fit in the time you set aside. Some patients cry as they tell their story. This is a normal response to relating an emotional experience, and it is not necessarily a reason to stop the interview unless the patient wants to stop. You should try to be supportive and say something like "It sounds like this was a very difficult experience for you (and your family). Do you want to go on or would you prefer to stop now?" Try to sit quietly when the patient is silently thinking about a response, and maintain eye contact if the patient shows emotion. Good eye contact and attention demonstrate appropriate respect for the patient's story.

✐ Sometimes the interview does not go well. It might be that the patient isn't feeling well enough to talk or they are taken away for a test in the middle of the conversation. Maybe they were up for most of the night or they are in pain and are feeling angry or irritable. The reality is that, in a busy hospital, there are likely to be a number of interruptions. Do the best that you can.

✐ Some patients are angry about the course of their life, the illness, or their medical care, and that anger may spill over into your interview. In this case, try asking an open-ended question like "What would you want the doctors to know about what it is like to live with illness?" If they still are angry or you feel uncomfortable, thank them for their time and excuse yourself.

✐ Some patients just won't talk – or at least they won't say anything with real content. It could be that they are just too exhausted. Others find it difficult to talk about personal or emotional issues. However, there is also a lot to be learned from what is not said. If you are interviewing a patient who tells you that life is fine, that their family is supportive, that there are no issues, and the interview seems to fall flat, you should think and write about why the person is responding in this way. They may simply feel uncomfortable discussing such personal things with you, they may not be a very reflective person, or they may not have dealt with a number of the issue that you are raising.

✐ When you have finished the interview, thank the patient for their time and for helping you to learn about the impact of illness. Let them know that their remarks have been helpful and that you will try to remember the issues they discussed as you care for patients in the future.

SUGGESTED QUESTIONS FOR PATIENT INTERVIEWS

Start the interview by introducing yourself and thanking the patient for taking time to talk to you. Tell them that you are trying to understand how illness effects people in their personal life – their sense of who they are, their relationships at home and at work, and their emotions. Then ask them if it is OK to interview them about these personal aspects of their illness. If they say yes, then here are some issues to talk about. Don't expect to cover all of them in one interview.

✏ How were you given the diagnosis? Do you remember your reaction?

✏ What was the impact of the illness on:
  — your self-image?
  — your relationships with friends?
  — your roles at home?
  — your relationships at home with partner and/or children?
  — your roles at work and your ability to work?
  — your relationships with co-workers and employers?

✏ If the patient is disabled, ask them how they feel about being out of work.

✏ Have you ever felt lonely or isolated because of the illness? Can you explain how you felt?

✏ What has helped you most to adjust to the illness?
  — The role of friends and family.
  — Other supports.
  — Religion and spirituality.
  — Other.

✏ What has been the most difficult part of adjusting to the illness?

✏ What aspects of your doctors' care have been most helpful and least helpful?

✏ Ask about the process of medical care
  — What has been most helpful and most frustrating?
  — How do you feel about hospitalization?
  — How do you feel about taking medications?

✏ Has the illness caused financial problems due to either the cost of medical care or loss of income? What was the impact of this?

✏ Did you notice any changes in their mood or emotional well being? (You may want to start by saying that you know that many people who have lived with serious illness have periods of anxiety and depression, and then ask if they have ever experienced these feelings.)

✏ You might conclude the interview by asking the following questions:
  — What is the one thing that you should try to do as a physician to help your patients live with a serious illness?

⌐ What advice would you give another person who had just been diagnosed with this illness?

Personal Essay on Living with Illness

Albert Einstein conducted "thought experiments" that led to some of his major discoveries – including the theory of relativity. He would sit quietly in a room for hours at a time imagining the outcome of certain experiments. To help you to "step into the shoes" of a person with a serious illness, you will conduct the following "thought experiment." Imagine that you were diagnosed with one of the following conditions (you can choose which one) during the first year of medical school. After reading the medical history, answer the following questions. (Some of your responses will be personal information, which you are not expected to share, but you should still carefully think through and write down your responses.)

1   After 3 months of weight loss, you are seen at the Student Health Services and a routine blood test reveals an elevated blood sugar of 393. Further outpatient testing confirms that you have type 1 diabetes, and you start treatment with insulin. Your blood sugars are difficult to control and you are hospitalized twice during the first year of medical school, once for an episode of low blood sugar that caused a seizure, and 3 months later for diabetic ketoacidosis. Six months into the illness, you start using an insulin pump. When you ask about the future, your physician is optimistic but discusses the possible long-term complications, including loss of kidney function, neuropathy, vision loss, and problems with accelerated cardiovascular disease.

2   After 3 months of unexplained fatigue, unusual rashes, early morning joint aching, episodes of chest pain, and purple discoloration of your fingers you are diagnosed with systemic lupus erythematosus. The initial blood tests show that you have lost about 20% of your kidney function. You are admitted to the hospital for a renal biopsy, and in the 24 hours after your surgery you develop shortness of breath and are diagnosed

with a small pulmonary embolism from which you recover quickly. Treatment with high dose-steroids, immunosuppressive medications, and anticoagulants is begun. The corticosteroid medication causes acne, a 20-lb weight gain in 3 months, and some insomnia and irritability. If you are a woman, your physician cautions you that you should stop all estrogen-containing contraception.

Your physician is optimistic about your long-term course, but warns you that this is a chronic illness and that there are likely to be periods when it is more active. Your doctor thinks that there is only a 10% chance of long-term kidney failure which would require dialysis or transplant, but that you are making antibodies that can cause pregnancy loss (if you are a woman), and that all pregnancies will have to be carefully planned.

3 After a flu-like illness, you develop right arm numbness and dysesthesias and left leg weakness that last for 6 weeks. You are having some difficulty concentrating in classes and you notice some emotional lability. You are referred to a neurologist, and an MRI of the brain and spinal cord shows areas of demyelination. You are admitted to the hospital and told that the results of the analysis of the spinal fluid and MRI suggest multiple sclerosis. You are treated with high doses of corticosteroids and the symptoms resolve over 2 weeks and you feel back to your normal self except for mild weakness in the leg that is only noticeable when you try to run or walk up stairs. Although you are feeling better, your physician tells you that the course of the disease is unpredictable and pregnancy may increase the risk of progression. Expensive intravenous treatments are suggested.

4 After spring break of your first year of medical school, you begin to have chronic diarrhea and notice blood in your bowel movements. You have occasional episodes of urgency, and once became incontinent of stool while out at a social function with friends. You are seen by your physician, who finds that you are anemic, and a colonoscopy and biopsy are diagnostic of Crohn's disease. You start treatment with high doses of corticosteroids and develop acne, a 20-lb weight gain, striae on your hips, and irritability and insomnia. Because it is difficult to control the flares of your Crohn's disease, you begin monthly IV treatments with a medication, which increases your risk of infection. You have a good response to treatment.

WRITING EXERCISE AND CLASS DISCUSSION

1 Why did you choose this particular illness?

2 Describe what you think the effect of your illness would be on your first year of medical school.
   a) Do you think you would take time off or drop out?
   b) What do you think the school would do to accommodate you?
   c) Would you discuss the diagnosis with your classmates? If so, who would you tell or not tell?
   d) If your diagnosis was public, what do you think the reaction of the other medical students would be?
   e) What kind of support would you expect from the students in general?

3 Do you think that your self-image would be changed by this diagnosis? If so, how?

4 Do you think the diagnosis would affect your relationship with your closest circle of friends? And with more casual friends? Knowing your friends, how do you think they would react to this illness? Describe their strengths and weaknesses in dealing with your illness.

5 Given your personality, what would be your greatest assets in dealing with this illness? What would be your greatest weaknesses or challenges?

6 Who would be with you if you had to be hospitalized? Who would you call for help?

7 Who would be your greatest sources of support – family and friends – in living with a chronic illness?

8 If you have a partner or are in a serious relationship, how do you think that this relationship would be changed by your illness?

9 If you had a flare of your illness during a third-year rotation that required you to miss a few days of work, how would you handle this with the supervising resident and attending during a clinical rotation?

10 If you are married, how do you think your marriage would be changed by this illness? If you are not married, do you think that your long-term plans for your personal life would be changed by this diagnosis? If so, how?

11 Do you think that your long-term plans for your professional goals would be changed by this diagnosis? If so, how?

12 As you imagine a life with chronic illness, what would you be most fearful of or worried about?

13 Do you think that your personality or your outlook on life would be changed by serious illness?

14 Can you think of reasons why an illness like this could be a positive experience for you?

15 What kind of a physician would you like to have? As you think about the doctors you have known, what characteristics would you be looking for in your doctor? Do you think that you will be the kind of doctor that you would like to have as your personal physician? Why or why not?

16 Your medications cost $20,000 per year. What is your co-pay on non-generic medication?

Class Paper

At the end of the seminar, you will write a 4-page paper (double spaced) that synthesizes the themes discussed during the course and in the readings with the comments of patients during the interviews. Possible topics include the following:

1 Reflections on physician–patient interactions (best and worst) that you have observed during training, and how the readings, discussions, or interviews helped you to understand those interactions.

2 Contrast/compare the impact of illness on the patients whom you interviewed and the authors of the articles or memoirs that you read during the course. Why do you think the experiences were similar or different?

3 What was the most surprising or most helpful information you found in the readings, interviews, and discussions? Has the way you look at the practice of medicine changed?

4 How will the way you practice medicine change, given what you have learned from the readings, interviews, and discussion?

If you can think of other areas that you would like to explore, suggest them to your group leader.

Index